Boudewyns, Patrick A., 1940
Flooding and implosive
therapy.

FLOODING AND IMPLOSIVE THERAPY

Direct Therapeutic Exposure in Clinical Practice

FLOODING AND IMPLOSIVE THERAPY

Direct Therapeutic Exposure in Clinical Practice

Patrick A. Boudewyns
Veterans Administration Medical Center and
Medical College of Georgia
Augusta, Georgia

and

Robert H. Shipley
Veterans Administration Medical Center and
Duke University Medical Center
Durham, North Carolina

Plenum Press • New York and London

Library of Congress Cataloging in Publication Data

Boudewyns, Patrick A., 1949–
Flooding and implosive therapy.

Bibliography: p.
Includes index.
1. Desensitization (Psychotherapy). 2. Behavior therapy. I. Shipley, Robert H., 1945–
. II. Title. [DNLM: 1. Behavior therapy. 2. Anxiety disorders—Therapy. WM 425 B784f]
RC489.D45B68 1983 616.89′142 83-2380
ISBN 0-306-41155-5

A Division of Plenum Publishing Corporation
233 Spring Street, New York, N.Y. 10013

Printed in the United States of America

To Mickey, Brian, Patrick, and Erin
P.A.B.

To my father, J.B., and Kim
R.H.S.

PREFACE

Behavior therapists often "desensitize" clients by exposing them to an anxiety-eliciting stimulus such as a phobic object. The premise is that repeated exposures will eventually reduce or extinguish the fear. This process is called *therapeutic exposure.* Many therapists would agree that therapeutic exposure is an effective treatment for several anxiety disorders. However, the "directness" with which therapeutic exposure should be encouraged for a client is much debated. Many feel that direct therapeutic exposure, more commonly known as *flooding* or *implosive therapy,* causes clients an excessive amount of anxiety, and may therefore produce long-lasting and harmful side effects. In response to these concerns, one well-known behavior therapy technique, systematic desensitization, was designed to expose clients to imagined fear stimuli slowly and under relaxing conditions so as not to elicit anxiety. In the first chapter of this book, we show that these concerns are based on false assumptions. When used properly, direct therapeutic exposure is not harmful.

In Chapters 2 and 3, we review the literature on the process and outcome of flooding and implosive therapy from a practical, clinical perspective. This literature shows that these treatments are effective and efficient for certain psychiatric disorders. In Chapter 4, we describe the treatments we offer our clients and show how learning theory can be used to help develop the procedure and content of therapy. Chapter 5 provides case examples with transcripts of typical therapy sessions.

This book can be used as a handbook for therapists or students. If used as a handbook, we strongly recommend that those not familiar with the theory and rationale read the book thoroughly and try not to learn the technique from the case examples alone. For example, some of the transcripts in Chapter 5 involve anger, violence, and/or sexual concerns; material that might be upsetting to anyone. However, as shown in Chapter 4, this material is highly idiosyncratic to the client. There is considerable method in what might at first appear to be madness.

Finally, one aim of this book is to dispel the common belief that therapists who use direct therapeutic exposure lack empathy and concern for their clients. In fact, because these treatments sometimes provoke anxiety, it is vitally important that the therapist convey support and empathy so that the client is motivated to continue in therapy.

We wish to thank several people who helped us in writing this book. First and foremost, we offer our gratitude to our teachers, Thomas Stampfl and Donald Levis. Next, we wish to thank Jeannine Wheless and T. John Rosen for their superb editing, and Kit Chappell, Gill Lunsford, Marge Miles, Amanda Darwin, Paulette Fulghum, and Joan Way for help in preparing the manuscript. Finally, we thank our clients who allowed us to learn from them.

PATRICK A. BOUDEWYNS
ROBERT H. SHIPLEY

CONTENTS

1

DIRECT THERAPEUTIC EXPOSURE

Johann Wolfgang von Goethe, the German author, suffered from intense fears of heights, diseased bodies, loud noises, and dark, lonely places. As a 20-year-old law student at the University of Strasberg, he decided to remedy these infirmities. In his autobiography (Goethe, 1770) he wrote:

> I ascended quite alone the highest pinnacle of the cathedral spire, and sat in the so-called neck under the knob or crown, as it is called, for a quarter of an hour, before I ventured to step out again into the open air, where, on standing on a platform, scarcely an ell square, without anything particular to hold on to, one sees before one the boundless land, while the nearest objects and ornaments conceal the church and everything on which and above which one stands. It is exactly as if one saw oneself carried up into the air in a balloon. Such anxiety and pain I repeated so often until the impression became quite different to me, and I have therefore derived great advantage from these practices in mountain travels and on geological studies, and on great buildings, where I have vied with the carpenters in running over the free-lying beams and the cornices of the building, and even in Rome, where one must run similar risks in order to obtain a nearer view of important works of art. (pp. 326–327)

Goethe used similar techniques to treat his other fears.

A contemporary story about one of our daughters (P.A.B.) demonstrates the same principle used by Goethe to reduce fear. By the time Erin was 3 years old, a parentally administered program of modeling and reinforcement had trained her to put her dirty clothes into the clothes chute. The chute, which was near the floor in the hallway just outside Erin's bedroom, delivered clothes to a basement hamper. On one cold, Iowa winter morning, while Erin was wearing her long-sleeved flannel nightgown with elastic bands at the wrists, she dutifully picked up her dirty clothes from her bedroom floor, opened the door to the clothes chute, and pitched them in. (Erin, now a teenager, has successfully extinguished this and many other learned neatness behaviors.) At this point, she abruptly moved away from the chute, yelled "Help!" and started to jump around in a panic. When asked what the trouble was, Erin (who has always had a flair for unconventional but accurate description) screamed, "Something is walking all over me!" and pointed to a moving lump near the elastic band of her nightgown on her right arm. Her father quickly grabbed her arm and lifted up the elastic to release a mouse that had apparently jumped into her nightgown from the open chute. The mouse ran back down the chute, and Erin, unhurt but still shaking, resolved never to go near the clothes chute again. one trial learning! Erin proved good to her word. For the next several days no amount of parental coaxing could get her near the chute.

Her response to this situation was understandable. Nevertheless, both Mom and Dad were (of course) in favor of her continuing with the learned dirty-clothes-disposal behavior. In an effort to reinstate the behavior, her psychologist dad designed a "therapy" program which included modeling and cognitive strategies. First, he caught the (or at least a) mouse, showed the trap with the dead animal in it to Erin, and explained that this meant the chute was now safe. Erin responded appropriately to the stimulus ("Yech"), but verbalized satisfaction that the nightgown intruder was dead. Next Dad took her to the clothes chute, opened it and invited her to use it. Erin started toward the chute, but quickly backed off. When asked about this response, she stated that, while she was convinced that the mouse was gone, her "tummy still jumped" when she got near the chute. Something more was needed. Dad then persuaded her to close her eyes and pretend that she had put her hand in the chute. She was able to do this several times. He then requested that she do the same thing "for real" *(in vivo)* while assuring her that, if she did this several times, her tummy would stop jumping. This reassurance was enough to get her trembling hand up to the open chute. After a number of "trials" Erin stated that she would use the chute, but did so with obvious caution for several days. Within a week, it appeared as if her fear had been eliminated.

Both of these anecdotes illustrate the subject of this book; the process of direct therapeutic exposure. We use *direct therapeutic exposure* as a generic term for a class of therapies, most commonly referred to as either *flooding* or *implosive therapy.*

The aims of this introductory chapter are to: (1) define the term *direct therapeutic exposure* and familiarize the reader with the several alternative terms that describe the different variations or types of therapeutic exposure, (primarily flooding and implosive therapy); (2) identify those disorders for which direct therapeutic exposure has been effective; and (3) show why many modern therapists falsely assume that direct therapeutic exposure is ineffective and/or dangerous.

What Is Direct Therapeutic Exposure?

Direct therapeutic exposure is defined as: *repeated or extended exposure, either in reality or in fantasy, to objectively harmless, but feared, stimuli for the purpose of reducing negative affect.* Note that this definition is operational. It avoids all theoretical constructs, such as extinction, habituation, or conditioned inhibition.

Direct therapeutic exposure has also been referred to as *nongraded exposure* (Marks, 1975). This term implies that therapeutic exposure may gradually (graded) occur or occur all at once (nongraded). The therapist may expose the client to the fear cue in small increments, as in systematic desensitization, or all at once, as in flooding or implosive therapy. The anecdote from Goethe's autobiography illustrates a nongraded procedure. Had Goethe used a graded strategy, he would have slowly ascended the spire, stopping at various points along the way until he became comfortable, and then would have moved on. Of course, this process would have taken much longer than the more direct technique he employed. In this book we choose to demonstrate the use of the more direct techniques, which we believe in most instances have been both more efficient and effective than the graded methods. The reader should be aware, however, that very often the "gradedness" of therapeutic exposure in clinical practice is determined by practical matters (client acceptance, client motivation, and therapist–time constraints) rather than by scientific considerations. Looked on in this way, graded and nongraded exposure can be conceptualized as two ends of a single continuum.

The terms *flooding, implosive therapy, implosion* and *response prevention* are the most often used words to describe the types of direct therapeutic exposure discussed in this book. Other terms with similar meanings include *detainment, forced reality testing, forced exposure, deconditioning, counter phobic treatment,* and *extinction therapy.* A number of authors (Baum, 1970; Baum & Poser, 1971; Boudewyns, 1975a; Levis & Hare, 1977; Marks, 1975) have suggested definitional refinements for these terms. In the remainder of this section we discuss and review these semantic considerations.

The term *flooding* started to appear in the clinical literature of the late 1960s, as used primarily by the Maudsley Hospital (London, England) group led by Isaac Marks, S. Rachman, and their associates and students. The initial usage, however, should probably be credited to Polin (1959) who used the term to describe a procedure in which the conditioned stimulus (CS) is presented to an organism for an extended period of time. The organism is allowed to make avoidance responses during the CS exposure but these responses do not terminate the CS. Another term, *response prevention* (Baum, 1970), is often considered synonymous with flooding. Technically, the procedure of flooding differs from that of response prevention since in the latter avoidance is not allowed. In clinical practice, anxiety-laden cues are presented to the client and avoidance responses are either blocked (i.e., response prevention) or rendered ineffective in terminating the cues (i.e., flooding). We follow traditional clinical usage in this book by referring to both response prevention and flooding as flooding techniques.

Flooding, then, refers to direct nongraded exposure of a client to objectively harmless fear cues. There is no requirement or implication that the client must respond to the flooding in any particular manner.

The terms for the other most common type of direct exposure technique, *implosive therapy* or *implosion,* first appeared in the literature in a book by Perry London (1964), although Thomas Stampfl, the originator of the therapy, had given several symposia on the technique prior to this. Stampfl began to develop the theory and technique of implosive therapy in the mid 1950s, but it was not until the mid 1960s that he and Donald Levis published the *Essentials of Implosion Therapy,* which described the process and theoretical basis of the treatment (Stampfl, 1961; Stampfl & Levis, 1966, 1967).

In order for treatment to be effective, Stampfl feels that the client must emotionally respond to the scenes or cues. He asserts that repeated exposure to the fear extinguishes the emotional response in accordance with Mowrer's two-factor theory (Mowrer, 1947; Stampfl & Levis, 1967). Also, Baum (1970) and Baum and Poser (1971) have pointed out that implosive therapy refers only to "flooding in imagination" and thus should not include *in vivo* flooding. This may be true in practice, but Stampfl's theory would not disallow "*in vivo* implosion," at least when presenting so-called symptom-contingent scenes or cues (see Chapter 4).

To distinguish flooding from implosive therapy, Levis and Hare (1977) have pointed out that flooding therapists use only "symptom-contingent" cues. Flooding therapists also do not expose clients to imaginal cues that theoretically could be associated with the fear cues through higher order conditioning or generalization. Whereas implosive therapy often involves routinely exposing clients to hypothetical fear cues selected from ten specific (didactic) areas of probable stress or conflict (see Chapter 4), flooding involves the exposure of clients to only those situations that the client reports as fear producing. In implosive therapy, imaginal scenes may include hypothesized and "psychodynamic" cues as well as other material thought relevant by the therapist. Levis and Hare (1977), therefore, see fantasy flooding as a kind of incomplete implosive therapy. Boudewyns (1975a) suggested that flooding is simply an operational term describing a specific therapeutic technique, whereas implosive therapy is a formalized process implying therapeutic content, client response, and a complex theoretical and clinical orientation as originally outlined by Stampfl and Levis (1967) and elaborated on in Chapter 4.

These semantic issues may seem trivial, but they have presented significant problems for therapists. For example, many studies designed to test the effects of implosive therapy have not done so. Instead, they have simply tested the effectiveness of flooding or nongraded exposure in reducing fear responses to very specific cues. Unfortunately, reviewers have assumed that such studies have a bearing on the effectiveness of all exposure techniques. This confusion was especially apparent in the early reviews by Ayers (1972), Frankel (1972), and Morganstern (1973).

For Which Disorders Is Direct Therapeutic Exposure Effective?

In a recent conference several leading behavior therapists and researchers (see Barlow & Wolfe, 1981) concluded that direct therapeutic exposure is the treatment of choice for phobias (including agoraphobia and obsessive-compulsive disorders). As will be shown in Chapters 2 and 3, exposure techniques have also been used successfully with a variety of other disorders. In spite of these successes, many therapists still appear reluctant to use direct exposure techniques because of a historically acquired "bad reputation." Authorities from several theoretical orientations seem to have agreed that direct exposure is (1) ineffective and in fact may even increase, rather than decrease, anxiety, and that (2) it can be harmful to the patient. The aim of the next section is to demonstrate that such attitudes were based on questionable assumptions that have since been shown to be inaccurate and therefore should no longer concern the practitioner.

Early False Assumptions Lead to Concerns about Effectiveness

Direct exposure procedures were among the first psychological treatments for psychiatric disorders. While still under the influence of Breuer, Freud recommended a treatment for hysterical neurosis that could now pass for flooding. In a paper describing a case of hysteria, Freud and Breuer (1863) wrote:

> The discovery that we made, at first to our own great surprise, was that when we had succeeded in bringing the exciting event to clear recollection, and had also succeeded in arousing with it the accompanying affect, and when the patient had related the occurrence in as detailed a manner as possible and had expressed his feeling in regard to it in words, that various hysterical symptoms disappeared at once, never to return. Recollection without affect is nearly always quite ineffective; the original psychical process must be repeated as vividly as possible and brought into *statum nascendi* and then talked out. (Riviere, 1953, p. 28)

Also, at about the same time, Delboeuf and Binet described similar therapies in French medical journals (see Riviere, 1953, p. 28, footnote 1).

Many of these early therapies, including the hypnotic technique of Mesmer and others, stressed the need for an emotional response in therapy; simply exposing clients to the fear cue was not sufficient. It was felt that therapy would only be effective when it produced *catharsis* or *abreaction*. In his early writings, Freud assumed that patients had built up the potential to react with emotion, and that the job of the therapist was to stimulate that response. Hypnosis, for example, was seen as helpful because it allowed the patient to suppress or ignore those learned inhibitions that blocked the response. Thus, the stimuli generating the emotional response (e.g., early memories, daydreams, phobic cues, etc.) were not as significant as the response itself. The stimulus simply helped to release affect. Nichols and Zax (1977) metaphorically called this the "tea kettle theory of catharsis." Perhaps the emphasis on the response, rather than the repeated exposure of fear cues, made these procedures less effective than they might have been. For example, it is doubtful that Freud exposed the client to the fear cues a sufficient number of times to bring about extinction of the emotional response. As discussed in Chapter 3, the only condition necessary (if not sufficient) for effective direct therapeutic exposure is multiple and (preferably) lengthy treatment exposures. Later, Freud concluded on purely theoretical grounds that simple abreaction was not sufficient to maintain therapeutic gains. Freud's terse dismissal of abreaction inhibited subsequent analysts from using this technique. Instead, they used the much less direct exposure method of free association. As Nichols and Zax point out, abreaction and the use of emotionality as a curative measure came to be associated with charlatans and faith healers. An exception was the use of abreaction for the treatment of war neurosis and/or traumatic neurosis of other origins (e.g., Grinker & Spiegel, 1945).

Similarly, in analogue research with animals, there were early indications that direct exposure might not be effective. Early studies by Solomon and his colleagues (Solomon, Kamin, & Wynne, 1953; Solomon & Wynne, 1954), found that dogs that had learned to avoid a conditional stimulus, after being trained with a strong electric shock as the unconditional stimulus, showed little or no evidence of extinction, even after "many" trials. Solomon and his colleagues concluded from these studies that avoidance behavior (such that might be seen in human phobics) was extremely resistant to extinction and that in some cases it may be inextinguishable if the avoidance behavior is based on intense and traumatically painful stimuli (Kimble, 1961, p. 280). Later, however, researchers found that anxiety and learned-avoidance behavior in animals can be easily extinguished by using the proper exposure methodology (Baum, 1966; Bersh & Keltz, 1971; Polin, 1959; Shipley, Mock, & Levis, 1971). Thus, with only meager evidence on the animal analogue level and no evidence from research with humans, several early influential writers and learning theorists (most notably Dollard & Miller, 1950; Kimble, 1961) were pessimistic about using exposure strategies. Dollard and Miller concluded:

> To summarize, in phobias the responses of avoidance and their reinforcement by a reduction in the strength of the fear is almost always quite clear. The origin of the drive of fear may be obvious or obscure; it often traces back to childhood conflict about sex and aggression. *Fear can be exceedingly resistant to extinction.* The more exact determination of the factors that affect this resistance is a problem with important therapeutic implications. (p. 163; italics added)

Kimble suggested that, although one therapeutic possibility might be simple exposure to cognitive representation of the fear cue, such a ploy on the part of the therapist would be difficult at best. Kimble warned:

> A therapist well knows, one implication of this procedure is that painful anxiety* must occur during therapy if a cure is to occur. This fact is responsible for the main practical problems which arise in psychotherapy. As we have seen, the patient goes to great lengths to prevent having such

---

*Falsely equating anxiety with pain is common. It is important not to confuse the two. They are quite different both as theoretical constructs and experientially.

> anxiety aroused in him. The learning theorists might also raise a question about this procedure on other grounds. *If it is correct that very traumatic anxiety is inextinguishable,* it would be impossible to eliminate certain conflicts by reducing the avoidance gradient. (p. 470; italics added)

Thus, early behavioral and psychodynamic theorists agreed that producing strong emotions via exposure to anxiety eliciting stimuli was impractical, probably ineffective, and possibly dangerous. These conclusions were reached despite the fact that the question had never been put to a direct experimental test with human subjects.

Concerns about Resensitization and/or the Incubation Effect

In the field of behavior therapy, the most noted critic of the use of direct therapeutic exposure has been Joseph Wolpe. Wolpe (1958) developed the theoretical construct of *reciprocal inhibition* to explain how anxiety was reduced through a form of graded exposure known as *systematic desensitization.* The term reciprocal inhibition was borrowed from Sherrington (1906), who coined the phrase to describe the coinhibiting effects of oppositional muscles. Specifically, the original usage described the suppression of one reflex by the occurrence of its paired opposite. For example, as the leg is extended a reflex action serves to relax the opposing tensor muscle and vice versa.

Similarly, the psychological concept of reciprocal inhibition holds that a form of counterconditioning accounts for the reduction of any conditioned emotional response to fear cues. Opposing responses, such as relaxation, sexual responsiveness or assertiveness, must be allowed to inhibit or compete with the anxiety response if anxiety is to be diminished. Further, Wolpe contended that these competing responses are weak compared to the autonomic response of anxiety. Thus, the fear cues must be presented in "small doses" in order to allow the relatively weak competing responses to inhibit the anxiety. In using graded exposure, a *hierarchy* of cues is developed (i.e., fear cues are presented to the client starting with the least and progressing to the most fear provoking) and a new conditioned response to each fear cue (e.g., relaxation) is formed. Anxiety is thereby weakened by a progressive exposure to the fear stimulus. One cannot be anxious and relaxed at the same time.

Wolpe's construct of reciprocal inhibition is similar, if not equivalent, to Hull's (1943) theoretical notion of how extinction of a conditioned response is brought about. But neither Hull's theory of extinction nor the concept of reciprocal inhibition has withstood empirical investigation. Simple extinction (repeated nonreinforced exposure) is now considered to provide the most parsimonious and empirically verifiable explanation for the effects of any exposure technique (graded or direct) (Wilson & Davison, 1971). In fact, any advantage that the slower systematic desensitization process might have over flooding would probably be because the so-called inhibiting responses, in some cases, may increase the time the anxious client remains exposed to the fear cues. The advantages are not because of any direct inhibiting action of the incompatible response (Lomont, 1965; Wilson, 1973; Wilson & Davison, 1971).

What appears more important than the concerns about effectiveness is Wolpe's warning that direct exposure can actually increase anxiety. He believes that if patients are exposed to the full force of the fear cue, the resulting anxiety may, through association, increase fear responses via classical conditioning. This process is called *resensitization.* Similarly, Eysenck (1968) has suggested that some clients, particularly highly emotional clients, may respond to direct exposure with a paradoxical increase or "incubation" in fear rather than with fear extinction. That such an increase in fear *can* occur has been documented in several human analogue studies, using normals as subjects (e.g., McCutcheon & Adams, 1975; Stone & Borkovec, 1975), although in at least one well-controlled trial it was not observed (Kaloupek, 1980). As reviewed in the chapter on analogue studies (Chapter 2), this paradoxical increase in arousal appears to result from the use of an excessively brief exposure time and may be only a transient, procedural artifact rather than an enduring exacerbation of anxiety. In any case, no incubation or resensitization effect has been documented with samples of clinic patients, although it is well established that longer exposure to the fear cue is significantly more effective than briefer exposures in reducing negative affect. Furthermore (as will be seen in Chapter 3), exposure treatment has *never* resulted in more detrimental effects than that of untreated controls. Concerns about incubation and resensitization appear premature and overblown when applied to "real" patients.

In summation, early reviewers of direct exposure techniques tended to be critical and have therefore contributed to the belief that direct exposure is ineffective (Ayers, 1972; Frankel, 1972; Morganstern, 1973). But more recent reviews (Levis & Hare, 1977; Marks, 1975; Marshall, Gauthier & Gordon, 1979) have concluded that direct exposure techniques are effective. Most likely, the discrepancy is due to the fact that early reviewers primarily examined the animal and human analogue studies conducted in the late 1960s and early 1970s, whereas more recent

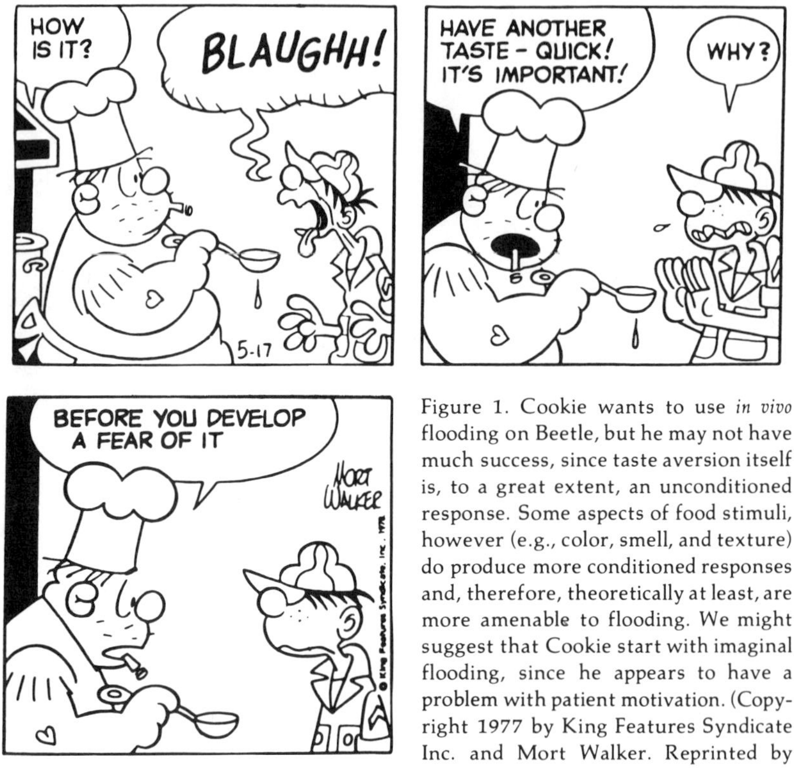
HOW IS IT?
BLAUGHH!
5-17
HAVE ANOTHER TASTE – QUICK! IT'S IMPORTANT!
WHY?
BEFORE YOU DEVELOP A FEAR OF IT
MORT WALKER

Figure 1. Cookie wants to use *in vivo* flooding on Beetle, but he may not have much success, since taste aversion itself is, to a great extent, an unconditioned response. Some aspects of food stimuli, however (e.g., color, smell, and texture) do produce more conditioned responses and, therefore, theoretically at least, are more amenable to flooding. We might suggest that Cookie start with imaginal flooding, since he appears to have a problem with patient motivation. (Copyright 1977 by King Features Syndicate Inc. and Mort Walker. Reprinted by permission.)

reviewers had the benefit of outcome studies on patient populations. Most of the results of the human analogue studies are greatly influenced by uncontrolled expectancy factors and demand characteristics. In light of the studies on expectancy and demand characteristics (e.g., Borkovec, 1973), the use of subclinical populations to support or refute the effectiveness of a treatment technique is not defensible. It is not clear why direct exposure techniques are more effective with clinical populations than with volunteers suffering from analogue fears such as snake phobias. One explanation might be that direct exposure therapy is most effective with problems, such as agoraphobia and obsessive-compulsive disorders, for which there is no true analogue population. We wish to make it clear that we *do* find that analogue studies are useful in a variety of ways; in particular, they help to elucidate general determinants of behavior change and help to generate hypotheses for clinical research. But they cannot be used to determine treatment effectiveness as used with clinical patients.

Does Direct Therapeutic Exposure Harm Clients?

Many clinicians fear that their clients will be harmed by the anxiety that is generated by direct therapeutic exposure. The concern is understandable; therapists have been trained to relieve anxiety, and provoking anxiety, even temporarily, seems inconsistent with this treatment goal. Psychoanalytically oriented therapists may contend, for instance, that clients with low ego strength could be overly stressed by any technique that produces high anxiety; "brittle egos" might "break" under the strain. Even behaviorists, such as Wolpe (1969), warn that in response to flooding treatment "some patients do strikingly well, others are unaffected, and some suffer exacerbations of their phobias" (p. 189). Wolpe further states that "to make a person worse . . . is such a dreadful experience that it does not seem justified to expose anybody to the possibility of it except in desperation" (p. 192). Others have stated that it may be overly tiring for the client to exhaust so many emotional reserves during therapy. For example, Morganstern (1973) writes "the emotional cost to the patient during treatment is an extremely important ethical consideration" (p. 381). And Nathan and Jackson (1976) suggest that "implosion therapy can be useful with phobic or anxious patients who can *withstand its rigors*" (p. 532; italics added).

Some textbooks advise caution in the use of exposure techniques (e.g., Bandura, 1969; Coleman, 1976). Singer (1974) refers to "the risk involved in the implosive approach" (p. 170). Rimm and Masters (1974) assert that, "the possibility of inadvertent sensitization and other potential ill effects, demands that the use of implosive therapy and flooding/response prevention be accompanied with caution" (p. 352).

In general, complaints about direct exposure techniques seem to be of three basic types:

1. Clients exposed to flooding or implosive therapy will be driven "over the brink" and become psychotic and/or violent, suicidal, or homicidal.
2. Direct exposure therapy will produce negative side effects.
3. The high emotion generated during exposure sessions will be hard on a client.

There is little empirical evidence to support any of these objections. In one experimental study designed to assess the validity of these concerns, Boudewyns and Levis (1975) subjected 24 low-ego–strength and 24 average-ego–strength psychiatric inpatients to repeated implosive scenes relevant to their own fears. By measuring physiological responses (heart rate and skin conductance level), low-ego–strength subjects showed less evidence of stress than did higher-ego–strength subjects during early therapy sessions when anxiety should be greatest. This suggests that low-ego–strength subjects were either unwilling or unable to expose themselves to the anxiety-eliciting cues. Results of pre-to-post therapy testing, self-report, and nursing report using an objective behavioral inventory indicated that no patient in this study went "over the brink" or showed increased psychotic symptomatology as a result of this exposure therapy.

We are not suggesting that these findings refute the hypothesis that low-ego–strength subjects are more prone to respond negatively to stress than normal subjects; given sufficient stress these patients may indeed show greater deterioration than normal subjects. It does indicate, however, that defenses of low-ego–strength patients are strong enough to withstand the rigors of at least imaginal implosive scenes.

In our clinical experience, no patient has been driven "over the brink" as a result of flooding or implosive therapy. What typically happens is that the client reports some increase in anxiety after the first therapy session and generally whenever new material is introduced, but anxiety is reduced during the next few sessions.

In order to check our experience with other therapists, we conducted a mail survey of psychotherapists who, either by virtue of the graduate school or internship program they attended, or as authors of articles related to flooding treatment both pro and con, might have been familiar with these procedures (Shipley & Boudewyns, 1980). Therapists were sent a letter asking if they had ever used implosive therapy, flooding, or similar direct exposure techniques. If so, they were asked to report (1) how many cases they had treated and (2) whether any "serious negative side effects," such as suicide attempts, acute psychotic breaks, physical illness, or violence, occurred, and, if so, in how many cases. They were also asked: "Compared to other treatments you used, have you found implosive or flooding treatments to produce more, the same number, or fewer negative side effects?"

A total of 132 letters were mailed. One hundred and nine (83%) were returned. Of these, 70 respondents indicated that they had used exposure techniques with a total of 3,493 clients (median = 24, range = 1–500).

Six respondents reported that "serious negative side effects" occurred in a total of nine clients (0.26% of the clients treated). Each of these respondents was interviewed by telephone to determine the nature and context of these adverse reactions.

In four of the cases (0.11% of those treated), the client suffered an acute psychotic reaction. Two of these were agoraphobic clients with histories of paranoid schizophrenia who were successfully treated with *in vivo* exposure but then became psychotic with paranoid ideation. In both cases the psychosis cleared rapidly with phenothiazine medication and did not require hospitalization; but the agoraphobic symptoms returned. The other two psychotic reactions occurred in young adults without a definite history of psychosis. However, both of these clients had presenting symptoms that, like the agoraphobics, might be viewed as protecting the client from close contact with other people. Again, both reconstituted rapidly with phenothiazine medications.

The remaining five clients showed an acute panic reaction during therapy sessions and/or increased anxiety between sessions. Three of these clients ultimately made a good response to therapy; one terminated therapy prematurely after a "flight into health" and one remained unchanged. In the latter case, a female presented with severe obsessive-compulsive symptoms. Following the initial session, the client became increasingly fearful and stated her belief that the therapist was trying to drive her crazy. After this, the therapist taught her relaxation training and initiated systematic desensitization. The client calmed somewhat but her original symptoms remained unchanged.

Finally, 13% of the therapists said exposure treatment produced more negative side effects than other treatments, 66% considered them equivalent to other treatments in the production of side effects, and 21% felt exposure treatments had fewer side effects. Stated another way, 87% of the therapists judged direct exposure to produce the same or fewer side effects compared to other forms of therapy they had used.

Since there were no control groups in the survey there is no way to determine whether the small number of negative side effects reported were actually the result of therapy or if they were inevitable. Yet, even if we assume that the treatments were responsible for the negative side effects, their low frequency and relatively benign nature are encouraging.

To summarize, neither the "over the brink" theory nor the concern that patients would suffer negative side effects received support from the survey result. No deaths or violence were reported. Acute psychotic reactions occurred in only four cases (0.11% of those treated). All involved paranoid ideation. In each case, alleviating the clients' presenting symptoms may have allowed increased contact with people that in turn may have precipitated the paranoid reactions. Of course, clients in any form of therapy can become violent, suicidal, homicidal or psychotic. In fact, a recent survey by Edinger and Jacobson (1982) suggests that training in progressive muscle relaxation is associated with psychotic symptoms in 0.3% of treated patients. Thus, there is no evidence that clients treated with direct exposure are particularly prone to these reactions.

The survey results do not speak directly to the presumed high emotional cost to the patient who is treated with exposure techniques. It is true that following a session of direct exposure therapy, the client generally feels tired or "wrung out." But the patient's anxiety level is usually lower after a session than prior to it. The concern for the emotional cost to the client may stem from the fact that the only experience many therapists have had with direct exposure therapy has been hearing or viewing "unfortunate" clients being bombarded with descriptions of terrifying scenes. Actually, direct exposure clients spend the majority of therapy time not anxious or, at least, not terrified. Initially, a relevant scene may produce great emotional discomfort, but the repetition of this material in therapy and in homework scenes rapidly diminishes the level of anxiety arousal. After a few presentations of the same scenes, it actually becomes difficult to elicit anxiety.

Most direct exposure therapists let their prospective clients know that such treatment will "require a lot of work on your part and a fair amount of emotional discomfort" (Shipley, 1979, p. 141). Clients generally view the temporary discomfort as minor in comparison to the day-to-day suffering for which they seek relief. In fact, dropout rates are low (Boudewyns & Wilson, 1972; Levis & Carrera, 1967).

In conclusion, direct therapeutic exposure is effective for several disorders. Furthermore, there is no evidence that exposure techniques are dangerous, or that they produce many negative side effects or that they exact a high emotional cost to the client.

In the review of the literature in the next two chapters, we have kept the semantic issues that were discussed earlier in mind; we have tried to identify each treatment reviewed by the most appropriate name (even when it differs from the name used previously). We have also separated analogue (basic animal and human volunteer) and clinical level studies because of our previously stated belief that the effectiveness of a therapy cannot be determined on the basis of analogue studies alone.

2

RESEARCH ON NONPATIENT POPULATIONS

Analogue studies of exposure therapies differ from the clinical situation in many respects. The populations (generally rats or college students) and problems studied (e.g., laboratory conditioned fears; small-animal fears) are not problems of interest to the clinician. In addition, analogue procedures, though similar to the clinical procedure on some dimension(s), still are vastly different from those used by the clinician. Clinicians often view analogue research, particularly animal studies, as having little relevance to the problems presented by their clients. Animal researchers note, on the other hand, that research on human neurotics is hopelessly confounded by the myriad sources of uncontrolled variation. They point out that the clinician is neither familiar with the client's specific conditioning history nor can he or she control it. In the middle of this argument stands the scientist who employs normal humans with "subclinical" phobias as subjects to receive treatment analogues.

Campbell and Stanley (1966) distinguish between the internal and external validity of a study. An experiment is internally valid if the independent variable is not confounded by uncontrolled sources of influence. Valid conclusions regarding the impact of the experimental manipulation on the dependent variables may then be drawn—but only for the population and situation actually employed in the study. External validity refers to the degree that the experimental results can be generalized to populations and situations other than those used in the research.

Animal analogue research tends to be high in internal validity due to the possibility of stricter experimental control of extraneous variables, but low in external validity when an attempt is made to generalize the findings to treatment procedures with human behavior disorders. Hence, behaviorists have been justly criticized by Berger and McGaugh

(1965) for uncritically assuming that findings from animal research apply to human situations. Investigations of therapy procedures with human clients have relatively little problem with external validity since they are dealing with the population and procedures of interest. Yet, because of the difficulties of achieving experimental control in clinical situations, internal validity is likely to be low.

Both animal researchers and clinicians have valid criticisms of the other's approach. Both have strengths and weaknesses and, we believe, contributions to make. We agree with Ford and Urban (1967) who have proposed a three-stage research strategy that begins with laboratory findings and proceeds to clinical practice. The first stage of investigation is basic research, generally with animals. The aim is to elucidate principles that are general (over and above any individual differences) through the use of contrived situations and controls so that only specific factors are varied.

The second or bridging stage of investigation involves taking the now elucidated research findings of Stage 1 and investigating their applicability to humans under restricted conditions. As in Stage 1, the investigation is as controlled as possible but, because of the limitations imposed by ethical and practical considerations, the degree of control is necessarily less. Yet this relative loss of control is offset by the closer approximation to the human situation of ultimate interest. This bridging stage, therefore, deals with the interaction of individual difference variables with experimentally manipulated variables.

In Stage 3, the principles and procedures investigated in the first two stages are applied to actual clients under relatively natural therapeutic conditions. Here the problem of generalizing across populations and situations, which is inherent in Stages 1 and 2, is absent. However, there are fewer possibilities for experimental control because practitioners cannot select the problem or the treatment procedure independent of the context within which they are working. They cannot treat any two patients precisely alike, and treatments across patients are, therefore, not strictly comparable. It is difficult in the clinical context to determine exactly which aspects of treatment are responsible for behavior change. Clinical research can test the overall efficacy of a treatment procedure (preferably a procedure developed on the basis of findings from Stages 1 and 2).

The three-stage research strategy is admittedly an over simplification. For instance, the division between human analogue research and clinical studies is frequently blurred, and as Kazdin (1978) has pointed out, all studies, including applied clinical trials, are analogues to one degree or another. In performing clinical research with client populations, the investigator changes the situation from what would exist in a pure treatment context. Thus, anytime an attempt is made to generalize from one situation to another, the likelihood of success depends on the degree of similarity on relevant dimensions. But, to date, most analogue fear research *has* differed from the clinical situation on relevant dimensions and is therefore of questionable value in the validation of treatment techniques.

The fact that the multistage research strategy recognizes that analogue research cannot generally *validate* clinical treatments appears to us as a proper admission (Cooper, Furst, & Bridger, 1969). It can help, however, to establish basic determinants of behavior, to develop hypotheses, to explain clinical results, and to clarify theoretical issues (Bandura, 1978; Goldstein, 1966; Levis, 1970). In keeping with this viewpoint, this chapter reviews the analogue literature under two headings: *animal analogue research* and *human analogue research*. Our aim is not an exhaustive review of the analogue literature. Instead, we will try to discuss issues that have been investigated by analogue researchers and to draw conclusions based on this research that might be of interest to the clinician.

Animal Analogue Research

An investigator wishing to perform analogue research relevant to the flooding treatment of human neurotics must pursue analogues of both neurosis and flooding. The search for a convincing animal analogue of human neurosis dates back to at least Pavlov (1927), who believed that the disruption of conditioned behavior patterns in laboratory dogs constituted "experimental neurosis." Due to the large animals utilized, sample sizes were necessarily small. Investigators soon began to use the laboratory rat so that larger numbers of subjects could be included in the experiment. This allowed for better control procedures and the use of statistical analysis of the data.

Procedures were developed that seemingly produced "neurotic" behavior in the rat. Maier (1939) used a blast of air as the aversive unconditioned stimulus (US). The resulting behavior included violent running and jumping, convulsions, tics, and finally passive or catatonic behavior. Later, however, it was discovered that the high-frequency sound generated by the air blast was causing audiogenic seizures and that the convulsions thus produced were not rodent analogues of the classical experimental neurosis (Broadhurst, 1960). Other attempts to produce experimental neuroses in rats employed conflict as the precipitating stressor (Bijou, 1951; Cook, 1939). However, Hunt and Brady (1955) found that rats "handle conflict . . . with aplomb," and Hunt (1964) later concluded that "the rat probably doesn't develop psychopathology of the extended sort seen among human beings."

With the benefit of hindsight, it appears that efforts to produce behavior breakdowns in animals that would be convincing analogues of human neurosis may have been misdirected. The attempts were predicated upon the assumptions that human neurosis is a discrete disease entity, that neurotic behavior is qualitatively different from normal behavior, and that it is governed by different laws than behavior in general. However, abnormal behaviors are increasingly being viewed as responses that follow the same "laws" of learning as normal behaviors. Therefore, efforts to produce convincing animal analogues of neurosis have been largely abandoned in favor of analogues of neurotic symptoms.

The Conditioned-Avoidance Response

Many investigators now view phobic symptoms in particular and neurotic symptons in general as conditioned-avoidance responses acquired in accordance with Mowrer's (1947) two-factor theory of avoidance behavior. Theoretically, two learning processes are involved in the acquisition of a conditioned-avoidance response (CAR). Fear is acquired through classical conditioning when a neutral stimulus is paired "in time" with a painful unconditional stimulus. The result of this association is that the originally neutral stimulus becomes a conditioned stimulus (CS) eliciting fear. This fear activates the organism to attempt various maneuvers in order to escape or terminate the CS. When a response is hit on that provides rapid escape from the CS (and thus avoids the aversive unconditioned stimulus), fear declines. This fear reduction provides (operant) reinforcement for the successful response, and the organism learns to use this avoidance response whenever confronted with the CS.

Animal analogue research on exposure treatments has typically employed a shuttle-box having a shock and a safe side, or a single compartment box having a shock grid and a safe ledge. A delay conditioning paradigm is used. The animal is presented with a "neutral" stimulus, such as a tone, followed several seconds later by a shock or other inherently aversive stimuli. When the rat moves into the safe position of the apparatus, the tone and shock terminate. After several such trials, the rat learns to move rapidly to the safe area when the tone is presented, thus avoiding the shock. The animal is then considered to have acquired a conditioned-avoidance response to the tone CS.

In extinction, the shock is disconnected and the tone is repeatedly presented. Typically, the animal gradually shows a reduction in avoidance responding. According to two-factor theory, this presentation of the CS without the shock results in Pavlovian extinction of the fear conditioned to the CS. Once divested of its fear-evoking potential, the CS can no longer provide the motivation and reinforcement necessary to maintain avoidance responding.

In certain situations, however, avoidance responding has been found to be highly resistant to experimental extinction (Brush, 1957; Levis, 1966; Solomon, Kamin, & Wynne, 1953). In an attempt to account for this finding, Solomon and Wynne (1954) proposed the principle of anxiety conservation as a supplement to the two-factor theory. They noted that, in the standard avoidance–extinction procedure, the duration of exposure to the CS in the absence of the shock is contingent on the subject's behavior, since an avoidance response terminates the CS. With a well-established avoidance response, a high rate of short-latency responses usually occurs.

According to the principle of anxiety conservation, short-latency avoidance responses preclude the build-up of much conditioned fear that, as an autonomic response, is presumed to have a relatively long latency. Thus, rapid avoidance has the effect of conserving fear and retarding fear extinction. Other investigators (Levis, 1966; Levis & Stampfl, 1972) do not view the latency of the fear response as crucial but feel that rapid-avoidance responses retard fear extinction simply by preventing much CS exposure and subsequent extinction on any given trial.

One logical way to hasten extinction of the fear response and the CAR it motivates is to expose the organism to the CS for an extended period of time in the absence of the shock (US). This has been done with animals through the use of a procedure called *response prevention*. A rat that has learned to fear a tone (CS) is forced to remain in the presence of the CS for an extended period of time by a physical barrier. The response–prevention procedure has generally proved effective in hastening avoidance extinction (Baum, 1966; Bersh & Keltz, 1971; Black, 1958; Carlson & Black, 1959; Hall, 1955; Lane, 1954; Nelson, 1966; Page, 1955; Page & Hall, 1953; Polin, 1959; Shipley, Mock, & Levis, 1971). This technique is considered to be an animal analogue of flooding treatment of fear-motivated symptoms in humans. According to two-factor theory, this forced CS exposure is an efficient way of extinguishing the fear of CS. Divested of the motivation of fear and the reinforcement of fear reduction, the animal stops avoiding the CS (i.e., extinguishes).

Page and his associates (Coulter, Riccio, & Page, 1969; Marrazo, Riccio, & Riley, 1974; Page, 1955) suggested that prevention of the avoidance response in rats facilitates avoidance extinction not through fear reduction but through the learning of a species-specific "freezing" or an immobility response that is incompatible with avoidance. The rat, unable to escape the CS, substitutes crouching and freezing to cope with the fear. In subsequent regular no-barrier extinction trials, the freezing response competes with the avoidance response and results in its extinction, despite the existence of high fear. However, multiple investigations have demonstrated that nonreinforced CS exposure during response prevention *does* result in extinction of fear (Bersh & Miller, 1975; Bersh & Paynter, 1972; Corriveau & Smith, 1978; Franchina, Hauser, & Agee, 1975; Linton, Riccio, Rohrbaugh, & Page, 1970; Morokoff & Timberlake, 1971; Monti & Smith, 1976; Nelson, 1969; Shipley *et al.*, 1971; Wilson, 1973).

Shipley *et al.* (1971) obtained objective measurements of the rat's activity level during response prevention. They found support for Page's assertion that rats are less active during response prevention, but this decreased activity did not negate the fear-reducing effects of the forced CS exposure. Response prevention, then, does reduce fear through CS exposure (Monti & Smith, 1976). Extinction of the "symptomatic" avoidance response is facilitated by this reduction in fear, but in the rat it may also be due to the learning of the competing response of freezing. Avoidance responding, as an operant behavior, may be influenced by many other variables such as frustration or intertrial interval cues (Brown & Jacobs, 1949; Morokoff & Timberlake, 1971). It is, therefore, not surprising that there is not a one-to-one correspondence between strength of fear and strength of avoidance (Kamin, Brimer, & Black, 1963). It cannot be assumed that extinction of fear necessarily results in complete cessation of avoidance responding or, conversely, that if avoidance has ceased, the organism has *no* remaining fear of the CS (Mineka, 1979; Testa, 1976).

Effect of Amount of CS Exposure during Extinction

The extinction of conditioned fear, like other classically conditioned responses, is a function of the number and duration of nonreinforced CS presentations. The more extinction trials, the greater the fear reduction (Kalish, 1954), and the longer the CS duration/trial, the greater the fear reduction (Murfin, 1954). It has been unclear, however, how number and duration of CS exposure interact in producing the reduction in conditioned fear. In the treatment of human fears, advocates of systematic desensitization utilize many brief exposures while flooding advocates administer fewer lengthy exposures.

In order to investigate the relative contribution of the number and duration of CS exposures, total CS exposure must be held constant while the number and duration of CS presentations are allowed to vary inversely. A number of investigators have done this but, unfortunately, they used an avoidance paradigm for fear acquisition and a response–prevention procedure to administer the extinction exposures. With these procedures, it is difficult to control the amount of fear conditioned to the CS since the subject's behavior determines the duration of the shock and the number of CS-shock pairings. The duration of (non-reinforced) CS exposure in the extinction phase is also, at least partially, determined by the subject. Furthermore, the number of trials to extinction of the avoidance response (the usual dependent measure) is probably a poor index of fear–response strength since it can be influenced by other variables. In light of these difficulties, it is not surprising that the findings of several studies that used an avoidance paradigm are contradictory. For example, when all groups received the same amount of total CS exposure across extinction trials, Polin (1959) found one long CS exposure more effective than several short exposures in extinguishing an avoidance response; Shearman (1970) and Schiff, Smith, and Prochaska (1972) found a single, long, CS exposure and several short exposures equally effective; and others (Berman & Katzev, 1972; Franchina, Agee, & Hauser, 1974) found a single long CS exposure less effective than many short exposures.

Shipley (1974) used Pavlovian acquisition and extinction procedures rather than an avoidance paradigm to investigate the question. Following fear acquisition trials, rats received CS extinction exposures for a total of 200, 400 or 800 sec. One-half of the number of rats received this CS exposure in 25-sec segments while the other half of the subjects received multiple 100-sec CS exposures. The rats were maintained on a water deprivation schedule throughout the study, and residual fear was assessed after the extinction trials by the amount of suppression of licking for water during a CS test probe. Extinction of fear proved to be a function of total nonreinforced CS exposure, irrespective of the number and duration of extinction exposures used to amass that total. Thus, 400 sec of CS exposure had about the same extinction effect, regardless of whether it was administered in 4 100-sec trials or 16 25-sec trials. The important variable was the total amount of CS exposure across trials. Similarly, Bankart and Elliot (1974), using suppression of eating as their fear index, found equivalent effects from a single 180-sec CS exposure and 18 10-sec exposures. Wallace and Scobie (1977) investigated this question using goldfish as subjects and employing an avoidance paradigm. They, too, found extinction dependent on total duration of CS exposure.*

This exposure variable appears to account for the majority of the variance in fear extinction. In two studies, Wilson (1973) found a high correlation between total amount of nonreinforced CS exposure and subsequent latency to reenter the shock compartment. After reviewing animal analogue studies of fear treatments, such as systematic desensitization, flooding, and modeling, Adams and Hughes (1976) concluded that "the most important variable appears to be duration of nonreinforced exposure to the aversive CS" (p. 233).

The effects of many variables on fear extinction have been studied. Investigators have explored the effects of the presence of food during extinction, of various drugs, of forcing the animal to move about, of graduating the stimulus exposure, of the presence of other organisms, and so on. However, in most cases, the effect of these other variables on fear extinction appears to be mediated by whether they increase or decrease duration of CS exposure. This general conclusion is consistent with the human research at the clinical level (see Chapter 3).

The Effect of Food

The presence of food during extinction exposure to the shock box has been found either to hasten or retard fear extinction, depending on whether the food results in more or less exposure to the conditioned fear cues. Thus, Nelson (1966) found that, when hungry rats were placed directly over a food dish in the shock compartment, they retained more fear of this compartment than rats placed in the compartment without the food present. When no food was present, the rats roamed around the shock compartment, receiving more CS exposure than rats rendered less mobile by the presence of food. A second study (Nelson, 1966) demonstrated that food facilitated fear extinction when the situation was arranged so that the food motivated the rats to receive more exposure to the shock compartment. This formulation is consistent with Wolpe's (1958) observation that food in the shock compartment was

*Unlike rats who may "freeze" when subjected to shock, the species-specific defense reaction of goldfish is likely an activity (flight-type) response. Because of this, trials to avoidance extinction in goldfish may be a more accurate indicator of fear–response strength than is avoidance extinction in rats.

more effective in reducing the fears in cats when "the pellets were tossed at widely distributed points than if they were confined to the food box" (p. 57).

Effects of Graded CS Exposure

The effects of graded CS exposure on fear extinction also appear to depend on the amount of total CS exposure received. Kimble and Kendall (1953) reported superior extinction with graded exposure to the CS. However, the subjects in the graded CS condition received much more CS exposure than the regular extinction subjects. When duration of CS exposure is equated, graduated and full-strength CS exposure has been found equally effective in reducing conditioned fear (Wilson, 1973).

Effect of Drugs

Nelson (1967) found that rats given the tranquilizer chlorpromazine showed less residual fear only if the drug resulted in greater CS exposure. Baum (1973) found that injections of chlorpromazine or the stimulant methylphenidate prior to response prevention had no effect on extinction rate. Kamano (1968) found no effect of the tranquilizer amobarbital on the effectiveness of flooding. In another study, Kamano (1972) found amobarbital diminished the effectiveness of flooding as did chlordiazepoxide.

In a large ($n = 406$) study, Taub, Taylor, Smith, Kelley, Becker, and Reid (1977) tested the effects of administering various doses of 10 drugs or combinations of drugs just prior to response prevention. In earlier studies (Christy & Reid, 1975; Cooper, Coon, Mejta, & Reid, 1974), small doses of amphetamine during RP had facilitated extinction of avoidance responding. However, the large Taub *et al.* (1977) study failed to confirm this effect, and they concluded that the earlier positive results occurred because amphetamine partially overcame the rat's tendency to "freeze" when fearful. Taub *et al.* concluded that "any beneficial effects of low doses of amphetamine are species specific." The administration of various drugs thought to have tranquilizing effects also failed to enhance the effectiveness of response prevention. These drugs included chlorpromazime, chlordiazepoxide, sodium amytal, meprobamate, physostigmine, ethanol, and morphine sulfate. Also, these investigators found (consistent with Baum, 1969 and Kamano, 1972) that heavy doses of some drugs (chlordiazepoxide and ethanol) reduced the effectiveness of response prevention.

Taub *et al.* did find that atropine enhanced the effectiveness of response prevention in facilitating CAR extinction. However, as these authors noted, because of the large number of drugs and dosages tested, some significant differences might be expected by chance alone. Other studies of atropine effects during response prevention are needed.

Effect of Forced Movement

Lederhendler and Baum (1970) found that mechanically forcing the fearful rats to move around the shock compartment during response prevention hastened extinction. They interpreted this as supporting the view that response prevention hastens extinction because it leads to the learning of relaxational responses to the CS. Actually, it may hasten extinction by forcing exposure to the grid and other components of the CS complex. Similarly, the facilitative effects of having a nonfearful animal present during response prevention (Baum, 1969), or of presenting distracting noises (Baum & Gordon, 1970), are probably also due to increased CS exposure.

Effect of Flooding to an "Irrelevant" Stimulus

Mineka (1976) found that flooding with an "irrelevant" stimulus sometimes boosted CAR extinction. After animals were conditioned to avoid both a tone CS in a jump-up avoidance box and a light CS in a shuttlebox, they were flooded with either the tone or the light in the appropriate avoidance box. All animals were then run to extinction in the shuttlebox. The animals that were flooded to the tone CS in a jump-box were labled an irrelevant flooding group since the extinction test took place to a light CS in a shuttlebox. These animals extinguished faster than nonflooded controls, with the relevant flooding group tending to extinguish still faster. This was interpreted as evidence for "trans-situational" flooding effects, probably based on generalization across CS modalities (light and tone). However, this interpretation fails to note that animals are conditioned to a CS complex that includes, but is not limited to, the discrete CS identified by the experimenter (McAlister & McAlister, 1971). Thus, the CS complex in the jump-up box included the tone, sounds and sights of ledge retraction, and the grid floor. The CS complex in the shuttlebox included the light and the grid floor. Extinction to one component of these CS complexes—the grid floor—could well explain the generalization of extinction effects. Viewed in this way, the flooding in the jump-up box was not irrelevant to flooding in the shuttlebox. The notion of "irrelevant" flooding effects is further weakened by Mineka's (1976) failure in a second study to find a facilitative effect when the "irrelevant" flooding was given in the shuttlebox and the avoidance extinction was tested in the jump-up box. In this study, only relevant flooding (in the jump-up box) bolstered subsequent CAR extinction in the jump-up box. There was no generalization of extinction across situations.

One interpretation of irrelevant flooding effects has been that any stressful procedure will enhance avoidance–response extinction through a generalized habituation to stress or some generalized stress innoculation effect. Baum and LeClerc (1974) found that 5 min of forced swimming (irrelevant stress) resulted in as large a reduction in subsequent avoidance responding when tested immediately as did 5 min of flooding. However, when the avoidance–extinction test followed the 5 min of flooding or forced swimming by 2 hr, only the flooding group showed an extinction effect. Thus, unrelated stress appears to produce an immediate but transitory effect. From this finding, we might conjecture that, on the clinical level, abreaction would have only a temporary ameliorative effect if elicited by irrelevant stimuli or stressors.

Serial CS and Resistance to Extinction

For most fear-conditioning studies at the animal level, the CS consists of one discrete stimulus (e.g., a tone) plus the contextual apparatus cues (grid floor, etc.). On the human level, the situation is often more complex with conditioning occurring to an array of stimuli. For example, a boy who is about to be spanked by his father experiences a sequential array of stimuli—seeing his father's angry face, hearing his loud angry voice, feeling the tight grip on his arm, feeling himself thrown over his father's knee, and then experiencing the sights and sounds as he feels the pain of the spanking. When paired repeatedly with the pain of the spanking, it is likely such a CS complex will come to elicit fear. Because it is a much more complex CS than is typically utilized in animal studies, the resulting conditioned fear may be more durable than has sometimes been found on the animal level.

Stampfl and Levis (1967) have postulated that a fear gradient exists across the CS–US interval, with those portions of the CS complex temporally closest to the US acquiring the most fear. Thus, in our spanking example, the boy feeling himself being thrown over his father's knee would elicit more fear than seeing his father's angry face. In attempting to extinguish conditioned fear, it would be best to present the entire CS complex (in the absence of the aversive US). However, if only a portion of the CS could be presented, presentation of that portion which was temporally closest to the aversive US should result in the greatest generalization of extinction effects. Boyd and Levis (1976) conditioned rats to avoid a three-component-serial CS consisting of (in order) a tone, white noise, and a buzzer. This series of stimuli was followed by a shock. Rats were then given forced exposure to one component of the serial CS—either the tone, the white noise, or the buzzer. All animals were then given avoidance–extinction trials using the entire serial CS complex. As expected, extinction exposure to the buzzer, which was the CS component immediately preceding the shock, resulted in faster extinction of avoidance responding than did exposure of the CS components more distant from the shock. Thus, extinction of fear is facilitated by presenting those stimuli most closely associated in time with the aversive stimulus. Of course, exposure to the entire CS complex remains the most desirable strategy.

Summary

It is inappropriate to cite analogue studies to validate a clinical treatment such as flooding. Analogue work is valuable, however, in identifying potentially important variables, and in predicting and explaining clinical results. Past efforts to establish convincing animal analogues of human neuroses have been largely abandoned in favor of analogues of neurotic symptoms. Conditioned avoidance responses are seen as analogues to neurotic symptoms. In theory, avoidance is learned according to two-factory theory. The animal learns to fear previously neutral stimuli, through classical conditioning, and then acquires operant responses to escape from the feared stimuli.

Extinction of the fear and (usually) of the avoidance responses can be accomplished by forcing the animal to experience the CS complex for an extended period of time. The longer the duration of nonreinforced CS exposure, the greater the fear reduction. Other manipulations (such as drugs) that have occasionally been found to facilitate extinction probably exert their effect by increasing the animal's exposure to the fear cues.

Exposure to irrelevant stressful stimuli appears to have, at best, only a temporary effect on responding. Thus, at least on the animal level, fear extinction is largely dependent on the duration of exposure to relevant feared stimuli.

What would we predict from the animal results about human results? Assuming common basic laws exist across species, extinction of conditioned fear in humans should be a function of the duration of nonreinforced exposure to relevant feared stimuli. However, just as the species-specific "freezing" reaction obscured this relationship in the rat for a time, species-specific human defensive maneuvers may obscure underlying relationships for humans. For example, humans can use mental mechanisms to avoid perception of relevant cues or stimuli. Also, just as animal avoidance–response strength has been proved not to have a one-to-one relationship to fear strength, it is not expected that human avoidance (symptom)–response strength will correspond exactly to fear intensity. Many operant influences, such as "secondary gain" from symptoms and demand characteristics of experiments, influence the strength of human neurotic symptoms. Other manipulations, such as drugs or homework assignments, would be expected to facilitate fear reduction to the extent that they increase exposure to fear cues.

Human Analogue Research

There has been great controversy over the proper role of human analogue research in the treatment of fears and phobias. Borkovec and O'Brien (1976) criticized the use of snake and other small animal phobics but concluded "one year from now (two, if we are lucky) outcome investigators will once again point out the fatal flaws inherent in our current methodology" (p. 168). They were "lucky"; two years later, Bandura (1978) strongly defended the validity and utility of the snake–phobia paradigm common in analogue fear research. Bandura (1978) highlighted the fact that the greater experimental control of analogue research makes it better able to identify specific determinants and processes of behavioral change. Thus, just as "airliners are built on aerodynamic principles developed largely in artificial wind tunnels" (p. 89), analogue–therapy research may tap the basic processes responsible for behavior change.

As stated in the introduction to this chapter, we agree that human analogue research has a significant role to play. It can form the essential bridge between basic animal analogue research and clinical research by elucidating general principles of behavior, generating hypotheses, and helping to explain clinical findings. But, just as wind tunnels cannot demonstrate that a particular airliner will actually fly, analogue research cannot validate a given treatment technique. Furthermore, certain attributes of most human analogue fear research, such as the common use of mildly fearful subjects who readily respond to the demand characteristics of an experiment, have compromised the ability of this type of research to perform even its appropriate functions.

The external validity of analogue fear research has been limited by the many differences between it and the clinical situation. Analogue subjects are typically college students who have expressed some level of fear on a questionnaire, evidenced by a refusal to approach a feared stimulus (generally a snake, rat, or spider) during a behavioral avoidance test. These subjects undoubtedly differ in many important respects from the patients a therapist would find seeking treatment. Most importantly, the intensity of their fear is generally much less than in the clinical population (Trudel, 1979). Small-animal fears may also differ qualitatively from the more complex neurotic problems presented in a therapy situation. They are, for example, less likely to be accompanied by the "free floating" anxiety, obsessional features, depression, general psychiatric symptomology, and disrupted social relationships that are common in agoraphobic and obsessive-compulsive disorders (Marks, 1975; Olley & McAllister, 1974). The effects of other nonproblematic differences, such as age, education, and occupation, between subject and client populations are unknown.

The context of treatment in analogue research is also vastly different from the treatment context in a clinical situation. College students volunteering to participate in a study (perhaps for course credit), who realize that they are in an experiment and have read an informed consent document and who are "treated" by graduate students, contrast sharply with the usual clinical situation of the client who seeks out a therapist of his choice and must pay for clinical treatment by an experienced therapist (Barrios, 1979).

To further undermine the generality of analogue findings, changes are made in the clinical treatment paradigm in order to facilitate experimental control. For example, analogue-implosive therapy may involve the presentation of standardized imagery scenes via tape recordings in contrast to the clinical practice of personal presentation of individualized scenes. As we shall discuss, the effects of some variations in clinical treatment procedures (e.g., the use of taped scene presentations) have been investigated, but their effects are still largely unknown. Generalizations to the clinical situation are therefore ill advised. In fact, generalizations to other analogue situations may be risky since subject and procedural characteristics differ greatly from one study to the next. For example, the selection of fearful subjects generally includes a behavioral-avoidance test with change in fear behavior later assessed by repeating this test. However, as discussed by Bernstein and Nietzel (1977), the great variability of test procedures limits the generalizability of findings. For example, instructions may be live, taped, or written; subjects may be strongly encouraged to approach as close as possible to the feared object or only asked to approach it as far as is comfortable. The experimenter may do anything from modeling the approach behavior to being entirely absent.

Borkovec and O'Brien (1976) have reviewed the evidence on several methodologic and target issues in analogue–therapy research that limits both internal and external validity. The demand characteristics of pretesting encourage subjects to overestimate their initial anxiety level (Bernstein, 1973; Borkovec & O'Brien, 1976; Trudel, 1979). Further, treatment is generally conducted under positive expectancy instructions that explicitly suggest improvement and that contrast with more neutral instructions generally given to no-treatment control subjects. Even in the absence of explicit positive expectancy instructions, typical therapy instructions are viewed by subjects as more credible than various placebo control instructions (Borkovec & Nau, 1972; Boudewyns & Borkovec, 1974; McGlynn & McDonell, 1974; Nau, Caputo, & Borkovec, 1974).

In analogue studies of exposure treatment, demand characteristics have proven to influence posttreatment approach behavior, particularly where weak subject-selection criteria were employed (Borkovec, 1973). This implies that the less phobic a subject is, the more his or her approach behavior will be influenced by the demand characteristics of an experiment. In fact, Trudel (1979) found that high-demand instructions influenced the performance of moderately (as compared to highly) fearful snake-phobic subjects on the more difficult Behavioral Approach Test (BAT) steps. Furthermore, physiological measures of arousal are much less subject to the distortion caused by such extraneous variables. For example, in snake phobics treated by exposure, Borkovec (1972, 1974) found that physiological indices of arousal were not influenced by positive expectancy instructions. Approach behavior, however, was strongly influenced by the expectancy manipulation.

One possible solution of these problems is to select target fears of more clinical relevance for analogue work. Borkovec and O'Brien (1976) review research that show fears of negative social evaluation (heterosexual anxiety, speech phobia) are associated with a much higher than average physiological arousal than are small-animal fears. Further research shows that social fears are largely uninfluenced by demand characteristics (Borkovec & Sides, 1979). Social phobias also have the advantage of being common both in the population-at-large and in the client population, thus facilitating subject acquisition and the generalization of research results (Borkovec & Rachman, 1979). Rosen (1975) has suggested that more highly phobic subjects can be obtained through newspaper announcements of subject need rather than through the undergraduate subject pool. In fact, he suggested "that journals accept studies employing mildly fearful analogue subjects only when authors of these studies document that they first attempted to recruit phobics whose relevance to clinical questions is clear" (p. 70). With the foregoing reservations in mind, human analogue research is reviewed below as it pertains to clinically relevant issues.

Duration of Exposure

Duration of exposure can refer to the duration of continuous exposure of a given stimulus presentation, to the total duration of exposure in a given session (i.e., number of exposure trials multiplied by duration of exposure on each trial), or to the total amount of exposure across all treatment sessions. Evidence from animal studies suggests that the variable of primary importance in fear extinction is the total duration of exposure to the conditioned stimulus complex. In general, fear extinction at the animal level has proven to be a function of the total duration of CS exposure, with long- and short-exposure trials equally effective when total exposure is held constant.

At the human analogue level, however, lengthy (massed) exposure has proven more effective than short (spaced) exposure, even with total exposure equated. Mathews and Shaw (1973), treating spider-phobic subjects, found massed (48 min) presentations more effective in reducing behavioral avoidance than spaced (6 8-min) presentations. Similarly, in an analogue study of systematic desensitization with snake-fearful subjects, Ross and Proctor (1973) found single lengthy exposures to hierarchy items to be more effective in reducing both behavioral avoidance and subjective reports of anxiety than an equivalent amount of exposure given in several brief presentations. In the treatment of public-speaking anxiety, Chaplin and Levine (1981) found scenes of 50-min duration produced less anxiety, as measured by self-report and observer ratings, than two 25-min presentations. Evidence reviewed in the next chapter points to a similar relationship in patient populations.

Some investigators have attempted to establish how much total exposure is required for extinction of fear. This question is difficult to answer since the amount of exposure required depends on the strength and breadth of the original fear conditioning. Mildly fearful analogue subjects should require less exposure than highly fearful patients. In their review of analogue studies, Levis and Hare (1977) note that positive results were generally obtained with a flooding procedure when a total duration of 100 min or more was used.

Fear Enhancement (Incubation) with Exposure

Eysenck (1968) has suggested that nonreinforced CS exposure may occasionally lead to a paradoxical increase (incubation) in fear, and that this phenomenon is most likely to occur in subjects high in anxiety/emotionality. Analogue studies confirm that fear may increase after brief exposure durations. Miller and Levis (1971) exposed snake-phobic students to a live snake for either 0, 15, 30, or 45 min. As is generally the case with analogue research (Trudel, 1979), all groups approached closer to the snake at posttest than they had at pretest. Yet subjects who had received 15 min of phobic exposure approached *less* than did subjects who received no phobic exposure. The 45-min exposure group did not differ from the 0 exposure group. This U-shaped approach function was replicated by Stone and Borkovec (1975) for subjects scoring high on a self-report measure of emotionality. The U-shaped function was also present in physiologic data when 15 min of exposure resulted in relatively greater anticipatory Galvanic skin response (GSR) and reactive heart rate than zero exposure. Furthermore, heart rate for the brief exposure group increased over baseline rate, which demonstrated an incubation of anxiety effect.

Marzillier, Carroll, and Newland (1979) had snake-phobic and nonphobic subjects imagine a snake scene for 15 10-sec trials (for a total of only 2.5 min of exposure). The phobic subjects reported an increase in fear and showed heart–rate acceleration over the trials. Nonphobic controls reported progressively less fear over the trials and showed a complicated heart–rate pattern consistent with orienting or attentional behavior.

McCutcheon and Adams (1975) selected female undergraduates who were afraid of viewing a film depicting surgery. In Experiment 1, subjects listened to a 20-min tape describing a surgical operation; all of these subjects exhibited increasing arousal as indicated by more GSR fluctuations. Later, on the behavioral-avoidance test, these same subjects failed to show improvement in coping with their anxiety and tended to have increased arousal. In a second experiment, similar subjects were exposed to 60 min of tape-presented material describing a surgical operation. As in Experiment 1, arousal increased for the first 20 min, but decreased thereafter. Subsequently, subjects in Experiment 2 could view more of a surgical film with less arousal, again demonstrating a U-shaped extinction function. Similarly, in a recent study, Chaplin and Levine (1981) found that subjects with a fear of public speaking who were exposed to 50 min of continuous fantasy flooding showed a U-shaped extinction function. Reported distress during the scene increased over the first 20–25 min and then decreased progressively thereafter.

Shipley, Butt, Horwitz, and Farbry (1978) prepared patients to experience the stressful medical procedure of endoscopy by having them view an explicit 18-min videotape of the examination either zero, one, or three times. While experiencing the actual endoscopy examination, patients who had viewed the videotape the most times were the least fearful as measured by heart rate, behavioral ratings, tranquilizer required, and self-report. This outcome supports duration of exposure as the crucial determinant of fear extinction or habituation. However, when subjects were classified as having either a repressing or sensitizing defensive style, a different pattern emerged for the heart–rate data. Sensitizers showed a monotonic decrease in heart rate with each additional tape exposure, whereas repressors showed an inverted U-shaped function, with one viewing of the tape producing the highest arousal. This U-shaped function in repressors is very similar to that obtained for GSR fluctuations by McCutcheon and Adams (1975), for behavioral avoidance by Miller and Levis (1971), and for heart rate and GSR by Stone and Borkovec (1975). Shipley *et al.* (1978) explained the U-shaped function obtained for repressors as resulting from a disruption of repressing defenses by one tape exposure followed by extinction of fear in those subjects receiving three tape exposures.

Kaloupek (1980) reports two studies of snake-phobic subjects. In one study, approach behavior proved a linear function of the amount of exposure to the snake with no indication of fear enhancement. In a second study, 0, 15, or 30 min of exposure to a snake were provided as a single (massed) exposure or as several (spaced) exposures. In the multiple-exposure condition, approach behavior again proved a direct function of total exposure duration. However, with a single massed exposure to the snake, the 15-min exposure group showed greater avoidance than the 0 exposure control group, replicating the fear enhancement effect. Apparently, some procedural differences determined whether approach behavior appeared as a linear function of exposure duration or as a U-shaped function. In the latter case, it *appears* that brief exposure renders the subject more fearful. Kaloupek (1980) posits two mechanisms to account for his discrepant findings and for the findings of fear enhancement by other investigators. First, on the basis of an unpublished literature review, he suggests that untreated control subjects show a *temporary* decrease in fear behavior 1–2 hours following conditioning or pretesting (similar to the "Kamin effect"). Exposure treatments disrupt this effect. The apparent increase in fear behavior following 15–20 min of exposure, obtained in several studies, would actually be due to a transient decrease in fear behavior in the control subjects. If true, follow-up avoidance testing several days after treatment should show a linear extinction function.

Second, exposure to the phobic stimulus may activate fearful memories concerning the phobic stimulus (Gordon, Smith, & Katz, 1979; Miller & Levis, 1971). The snake-phobic subject in a behavioral-avoidance test is then confronted not only with a snake but with the redintegration of past fear-eliciting thoughts and images regarding snakes. The subject is thus confronted with a compound CS composed variously of the nominal fear stimulus (snake) and the memories elicited by that stimulus. The observed increase in fear with brief exposures is then hypothesized to be due to an increase in the number of fear-inducing cues rather than fear enhancement *per se*. Additional exposure serves to extinguish fear of the phobic object and the associated cognitive cues it elicits.

In order to explain why the exposure of control subjects during a posttreatment BAT does not elicit increased fear due to fearful memories, it is necessary to assume further that subjects are able to suppress or otherwise defend against fearful memories during the single brief exposure. Thus, three stages are hypothesized. During initial exposure to the phobic object, the subject successfully defends against the redintegration of associated fearful thoughts and images, but with further exposure (15–20 min) this defense breaks down and fearful memories cause an increase in level of fear. Finally, with even more exposure, the extinction effect that has been ongoing from the start becomes dominant and decreased fear results. This is obviously a complicated set of hypotheses that encompasses internal stimuli and multiple-interacting processes over time. However, the two explanations offered by Kaloupek hold promise, either together or separately, for resolving inconsistencies between different human analogue studies and between findings in animals and humans. They deserve research evaluation. Unlike Eysenck's notion of fear incubation, these explanations do not imply any enduring ill effects because of brief exposure.

Whether fear enhancement occurs may depend on individual difference factors (e.g., level of emotionality, use of repressing defenses) and on procedural variations as to how and when the exposure is administered. Further parametric research is needed to sort out these factors. Yet, regardless of the mechanisms involved, it is clear that confrontations with fear-inducing stimuli *may* result in increased fear followed (with continued exposure) by decreased fear. Other individuals will show a simple direct decrease in fear as a function of the amount of exposure. In either case, it is important to continue exposure until fear extinction is observed. In implosive therapy, exposure duration is not set *a priori*. Exposure continues within and across sessions until the client no longer appears to be anxious. This practice is supported by findings from analogue studies.

Gauthier and Marshall (1977) investigated the efficacy of different criteria for termination of phobic stimuli. Snake-phobic female undergraduate students were exposed to a color film of a snake during three treatment sessions. Termination of film exposure was dependent on a reduction in heart–rate variability to baseline range, the subject signaling that she was no longer fearful, or two observers both signaling that the subject was no longer fearful. On a subsequent behavioral-avoidance test, the observer-determined duration subjects increased their approach to the snake the most, followed by the subjective-determined duration group, and then the heart–rate criterion group. This finding supports the common clinical practice of continuing exposure to phobic stimuli until the therapist judges that the client is no longer anxious. It should be pointed out, however, that use of the heart–rate variability criterion in the Gauthier and Marshall (1977) study resulted in less total exposure (46 min) than the use of the subjective or observer criteria (74 and 60 min, respectively). This may have compromised its effectiveness, and it is possible that use of a more stringent physiological criterion (e.g., heart rate varying below baseline or at baseline for X min) would increase effectiveness. Hughes, Holder, and Dubois (1978), on the other hand, used yoked controls to hold CS exposure constant and still found individualized exposure durations most effective in reducing avoidance responding.

Mode of Cue Presentation

Fear cues may be presented to the subject in fantasy, *in vivo*, or pictorially through the use of slides or videotape. In each case, it is possible for the therapist to be present or absent during exposure. Review of analogue comparisons between *in vivo* exposure and fantasy exposure support the conclusion that, while both may be helpful, *in vivo* exposure is the more powerful (Marks, 1975; Marshall, Gauthier, & Gordon, 1979). However, many analogue studies have used tape-recorded imagery scenes because they facilitate standardization and economy of treatment. Levis and Hare (1977) note that this violates implosive-therapy procedures in two ways. First, the cues that are presented are not individualized according to the specific subject, nor can they be modified based on the subject's response. Second, the subject may block out or otherwise avoid a tape-recorded scene more easily than a stimulus presented by a therapist. Each of these possibilities, the presentation of the wrong cues or subject avoidance of the right cues, would result in less relevant exposure and less extinction of fear. Indeed, reviews of analogue studies find that the use of taped scenes has been more often associated with negative outcomes than has the use of scenes presented live (Levis & Hare, 1977; Marks, 1975). However, many studies have obtained positive results using taped scenes, which suggests that taped cue presentation can be effective. The conditions moderating its effectiveness remain to be investigated.

Sherry and Levine (1980), in the only study to compare different methods of scene presentation (taped versus live versus slide) in comparable (speech phobic) subjects, found therapist presence to be the critical variable. In this study, both live and taped presentations produced equivalent results if a therapist was present during the session. Slides failed to enhance the effectiveness of exposure scenes. Sherry and Levine interpret their results as support for Wolpe's (1969) contention that the therapist's presence induces relaxation which in turn inhibits anxiety. Noting that research shows relaxation unnecessary in systematic desensitization (e.g., Marks, 1975), a better interpretation may be that the therapist's presence facilitated increased exposure to the scene. Student volunteers may simply be more attentive to scene material when the experimenter/therapist is present.

It is important to note that all the flooding treatments in the Sherry and Levine (1980) study were associated with a decrease in speech anxiety when compared to no-treatment wait-list controls. This suggests that taped scenes can be effective. As used clinically, implosive homework scenes may be presented via a tape (of a scene presented in a prior therapy session) or simply imagined by the client without any outside aides. Clients generally report that homework scenes produce anxiety, but of less magnitude than the live scenes presented during therapy sessions. It is believed that if the homework scenes generate anxiety—indicating that relevant material is being presented—they will facilitate the extinction process. This supposition has not been subjected to empirical test.

In Vivo versus Fantasy Exposure

Reviews of analogue comparisons between *in vivo* exposure and exposure in imagery to feared stimuli support the conclusion that exposure is more effective when presented *in vivo* (Marks, 1975; Marshall, Gauthier, & Gordon, 1979). It makes sense from a theoretical standpoint that actual exposure to a feared stimulus complex would generate a more rapid extinction than fantasy exposure, since the latter is further removed on the generalization of extinction gradient then the former. However, some stimuli present during fear conditioning and can only be presented in fantasy. Other complex fear cues, as for instance a patient who fears disease or death, preclude repeated *in vivo* exposure. In the clinical context, where *in vivo* and fantasy exposure have proven effective, there may be no need to pick one type over the other. Typically, both fantasy and real-life exposure are employed.

The Validity of Using Imagery in Direct Exposure Techniques

The use of imagery in fantasy flooding and implosive therapy is based on the hypothesis that images and overt stimuli are to some extent functionally equivalent (Bandura, 1969; Cautela & Baron, 1977; Strosahl & Ascough, 1981). Specifically, it is assumed that (1) an image of a feared object or situation will elicit fear in a similar fashion to the actual object or situation and (2) this fear can be extinguished through repeated exposure as when the fear is elicited by the direct perception of external stimuli. A series of studies by Shepard (1978) and his colleagues have shown that imagery and direct perception, in fact, have much in common. For example, in reaction–time experiments, the imagining of an object or operation elicited a yes-no judgment in approximately the same amount of time as did a direct perception. Physiological arousal has been found to be greater while imagining a fear stimulus than while imagining a neutral stimulus. In fact, the arousal experienced through imagining approaches the arousal experienced when confronted with the actual stimulus (May, 1977 a, b; Van Egeren, Feather, & Hein, 1971). The degree of increase in physiologic arousal elicited by a fearful image is proportional to the reported vividness of the image (Drummon, White, & Ashton, 1978; Lang, Melamed, & Hart, 1978; Rimm & Bottrell, 1969). There is also evidence that suggests people can learn to produce more vivid imagery through practice (May, 1977a; Strosahl & Ascough, 1981). As to the second question, accumulated evidence suggests that fear associated with images and thoughts is subject to habituation and extinction with repetition (e.g., Parkinson & Rachman, 1980; Waters & McDonald, 1973).

A further issue in establishing imagery as a technique in direct-exposure therapy concerns what the elements of an image should be. Images may incorporate only stimulus characteristics (e.g., "See the snake"), response characteristics (e.g., "Your heart is racing, you can't run"), or both. Lang (1977) divides the response elements of the image into three classes (verbal, overt behavior, and physiological response). He contends that in systematic desensitization the therapist's description primarily includes stimulus descriptions ("propositions"). During flooding imagery instructions are primarily response propositions (though he notes that stimulus descriptors are also included). Lang believes that images which include both stimulus and response descriptions will produce more vidid imagery, cause a greater affect, and hence greater therapeutic changes.

Lang's view emphasizes that it may be fruitful to think of images not just as cognitive "pictures" of overt conditioned stimuli, but also as including various response elements. This view is consistent with Stampfl's theory of implosive therapy. In implosive therapy, many response elements (e.g., a racing heart) also serve as conditioned stimuli for further emotion. According to Stampfl and Levis (1967), it is essential that these elements be included in imagery so that the emotional loading of the images may extinguish.

Despite the evidence supporting the importance of imagery, research has yet to establish any relationship between imagery characteristics and therapy outcome (e.g., McLemore, 1972). It is not clear whether therapeutic outcome is actually independent of imagery ability or whether our measurement techniques and research methodology have been inadequate to uncover a relationship (Strosahl & Ascough, 1981). Many quesionnaire measures of imagery are available (e.g., Gordon, 1949; Hiscock, 1978; Sheehan, 1967). Most instruments, however, fail to recognize that imagery ability is probably not a unitary trait. Some individuals can imagine certain response modalities (e.g., behavioral avoidance) better than other modalities (e.g., heart–rate acceleration). Similarly, individuals may possess more or less imagery ability in different sense modalities or along disparate imagery dimensions. Given this, future imagery–measurement instruments might well be multidimensional. An imagery questionnaire by Switras (1978) has much to recommend it along these lines. Seven sensory modalities are measured along the dimensions of vividness and controllability, as well as providing two parallel test forms as a research aid. To date, no established questionnaire addresses the fact that image clarity is often adversely affected by negative emotions (Haney & Euse, 1976; Strosahl & Ascough, 1981). In exposure treatments, the individual's ability to use imagery while highly aroused may be more relevant than the patient's general imagery abilities.

Scene Content

Probably the most controversial aspect of implosive therapy has been the inclusion of scene content that goes beyond the concrete fear–stimulus complex. Snake phobics should imagine a snake, but why should they imagine the snake biting them or, based on psychodynamic theory, imagine a penis? Stampfl and Levis (1967) refer to the concrete stimuli (snakes) as "symptom-contingent cues", or those external stimuli that directly elicit symptoms. Thoughts and images initiated by the concrete stimuli are referred to by Stampfl and Levis as "hypothesized sequential cues" and have been variously described by others as "horrifying" or "unrealistic" (Morganstern, 1973). In the case of snake phobics, the subject may fear bodily injury and/or death through a snake bite, or, if looked at in psychodynamic terms, the snake may itself be a generalized fear stimulus with the primary fear object being the penis.

At the clinical level, the goal is always to hypothesize what stimulus complex the client is avoiding, including external and internal stimuli. This is done through intensive interview, observation, and the therapist's past experience. Even where horrifying or psychodynamic material are thought to be part of the feared stimulus complex, the therapist would generally first present the symptom-contingent cues. If repetition of these cues prove sufficient to relieve the problem, fine. If not, hypothesized cues are presented and their relevance judged by the client's reaction to them. Client improvement following presentation of symptom-contingent cues is most likely to occur with uncomplicated simple phobias, particularly if they are of relative low intensity (e.g., analogue small-animal phobias). In the interest of greater specificity and to stimulate research, Stampfl (1970) presented four cue categories and Levis and Hare (1977) seven categories. Both systems are discussed in Chapter 4.

Much of the analogue work on scene content has compared the presentation of symptom-contingent cues (flooding) with the presentation of hypothesized cues, with the latter identified as an analogue of implosion. In practice, implosion may employ *both* types of cues and never uses hypothesized cues without symptom-contingent cues. Further, cue material in analogue studies has not been individualized. For example, it is assumed that all rat phobics fear being bitten (e.g., Foa, Blau, Prout, & Latimer, 1977). Finally, it is frequently unclear why particular cues are hypothesized to relate to particular fears. Levis and Hare (1977) questioned the relevance of the scenes used by Fazio (1970) (involving loss of control, aggression, etc.) to the treatment of subjects who are fearful of cockroaches. Given these problems, it is surprising that some studies have found presentation of hypothesized cues equivalent to presentation of symptom-contingent cues in therapeutic effect (Foa *et al.*, 1977; Prochaska, 1971). However, in these studies, like others on this issue, methodological problems make conclusions premature.

What is needed are studies that compare the presentation of

symptom-contingent cues alone to the presentation of symptom-contingent cues combined with individually prescribed hypothesized cues. The exact type of cues presented should be carefully described in all research reports.

Flooding versus Systematic Desensitization

A popular study design, particularly in accomplishing a doctoral dissertation, has been the comparison of analogue flooding to analogue desensitization. Reviews have noted the preponderance of poorly designed studies and the variability in outcome (Levis & Hare, 1977; Marks, 1975). Such analogue comparisons are fraught with difficulties. Subject selection, treatment procedures, and treatment agent all generally differ from the clinical situation and, as happens in these poorly designed studies, basic boundary conditions of each treatment are violated.

Another problem with these types of "horse race" studies is that both treatments involve fantasy exposure to relevant fear cues. As we have previously noted, extinction of fear at the infrahuman level appears to be a function of the total amount of exposure to the nonreinforced CS complex. Given this, it would be important to control exposure time in treatment comparisons. When exposure time has been equated, no differences have been found between the two treatments (Mylar & Clement, 1972).

Effect of Drugs

At the human analogue level, little research has been conducted on the influence of the addition of drugs to flooding. In two small-sample studies, Whitehead and his colleagues have found that diazepam facilitated flooding (Whitehead, Blackwell, & Robinson, 1978) and that it had no effect (Whitehead, Robinson, Blackwell, & Stutz, 1978). It is our guess that drug effects are mediated by whether the particular drug regimen and time of administration facilitates or hampers the necessary exposure to feared cues.

Summary

Although human analogue research is ill suited to validate a treatment technique for patient use, it can appropriately be used to generate hypotheses, elucidate general principles of behavior, and explain clinical findings. However, human analogue fear research has been hampered in performing these legitimate functions by the use of mildly fearful subjects who respond readily to the demand characteristics of an experiment. It has been suggested that future analogue research use highly fearful subjects with clinically relevent fears (for instance, speech phobia).

Findings at the human analogue level suggest that lengthy (massed) exposure is more effective than short (spaced) exposure, even when total exposure is equal. The amount of total exposure required for fear extinction is likely to depend on the strength of the original fear conditioning, but positive results have rarely been obtained with total exposure durations of less than 100 minutes. Analogue studies show that fear *may* increase after brief exposures to fear cues, but then decreases with continued exposure to these cues. This may be due to procedural artifacts or to the activation of fearful memories that increase the pool of fear-inducing stimuli. Analogue research has supported the clinical practice of continuing exposure to fear cues until observation suggests that the subject is no longer fearful.

Fear cues may be presented *in vivo*, in imagery, or pictorially. In each case, the therapist may be present or absent during such exposure. However, imagery exposure is most effective when administered in the therapist's presence. Basic research on imagery supports its use as a "stand in" for real life stimuli yet analogue research suggests that, while any mode of stimulus presentation may be effective in reducing fear, *in vivo* exposure is the most effective. Nonetheless, physiological arousal while imagining a fear stimulus has been found to approximate that experienced with an actual fear stimulus. The degree of arousal is proportionate to the reported vividness of the imagery. As with real life stimuli, fear associated with images is subject to extinction with repetition. Despite these findings, research has yet to establish any relationships between imagery characteristics and therapy outcome. Further research with better imagery measures is needed.

Research on the effect of including hypothesized cue material in fantasy stimulus scenes has been fraught with so many methodological and theoretical weaknesses that even tentative conclusions are premature. Studies are needed which compare the presentation of symptom-contingent cues alone (fantasy flooding) to the presentation of these cues, plus individually prescribed hypothesized cues (implosive therapy). Similarly, analogue comparisons of flooding with systematic desensitization have been problematic and no conclusions are possible.

3

RESEARCH ON PATIENT POPULATIONS

Exposure techniques have been most effective with anxiety-based disorders, especially those types of anxiety disorders for which the anxiety becomes associated with either an external stimulus, such as a phobic object, or an internal stimulus, such as an obsessive thought. Researchers have also evaluated the effects of exposure techniques applied to several other diagnoses not strictly classified as anxiety disorders but which often have an anxiety component. These include alcoholism, agitated depression, psychosis, and insomnia. In this chapter we review the studies on client samples that have addressed the issues of interest to the practicing clinician.

Issues in the Treatment of Anxiety Disorders with Therapeutic Exposure

In Vivo versus Imaginal (Fantasy) Exposure

Although many studies have found imaginal and/or *in vivo* exposure to be effective treatments for a variety of disorders (e.g., Boudewyns & Wilson, 1972; Boudewyns, 1975; Boulougouris, Marks, & Marset, 1971; Hogan, 1966; Levis & Carrera, 1967; Mathews, Teasdale, Munby, Johnston, & Shaw, 1977), controversy over the *relative* effectiveness of these procedures is still alive. Similar to the outcomes from human analogue studies, the clinical studies reviewed below generally find *in vivo* exposure to be more effective than fantasy exposure, at least in the short run. However, recent clinical studies suggest that the combining of imaginal exposure with *in vivo* exposure may be the most effective way to *maintain* clinical improvement.

In an early study, Watson, Gaind, and Marks (1971) reported that 8 of 10 phobics treated with imaginal flooding followed by *in vivo* flooding were "greatly helped." Outcome measures included heart rate changes before, during, and after exposure to the feared cues, a patient–change score, and a clinical rating measure designed to assess fear experience on a 10-point scale. However, Watson *et al.* also reported that *in vivo* experience was more effective than imaginal flooding. Two other crossover studies of agoraphobics (Stern & Marks, 1973; Watson, Mullett, & Pillay, 1973) also found *in vivo* exposure to be superior to imaginal flooding.

In a large and well-controlled study, Emmelkamp and Wessels (1975) compared two groups of agoraphobics ($n = 19$) treated with four 90-min sessions of flooding. One group had a prolonged exposure *in vivo* while the other received flooding in imagination. A third group was given four sessions of combined *in vivo* and imaginal flooding (45 min for each method). Following the first four sessions, psychological tests, self-reports, independent observations, and *in vivo* measurements were used to evaluate progress. At this point, the group that received *in vivo* exposure only appeared to have benefited most from treatment. The combined *in vivo* and imaginal group also improved significantly but somewhat less than the *in vivo* group. Least affected by the treatment was the imaginal group. Long-term effects of treatment could not be assessed because all subjects were eventually treated with 10 sessions of *in vivo* flooding, the last eight of which were carried out as homework assignments with very little therapist contact. Two other similar studies by Emmelkamp and colleagues (Emmelkamp, 1974; Everaerd, Rijken, & Emmelkamp, 1973) also supported the conclusion that imaginal exposure did not enhance the effect of *in vivo* treatment.

In a well-controlled study, Mathews, Johnston, Lancashire, Munby, Shaw, and Gelder (1976) compared the effects of imaginal flooding to *in vivo* exposure in the treatment of 36 agoraphobics. The sample was divided into three equal groups. One received eight 90-min sessions of imaginal flooding followed by eight 90-min *in vivo* practice sessions. The second received 16 sessions (45 min of each procedure during each session) of combined imaginal flooding and *in vivo* practice. The third group was given 16 *in vivo* practice sessions alone. Symptom ratings, psychometric tests, psychological records, and behavioral measurements were collected after 8 sessions, 16 sessions, and again at a 16-month follow-up. The authors concluded that there were no significant differences among the treatment groups, although there was some evidence that subjects' responses varied according to the therapist by whom they were treated, regardless of the treatment group.

In a "reanalysis" of these data, Johnston, Lancashire, Mathews, Munby, Shaw, and Gelder (1976) reported that measures of effects immediately following therapy indicated that imaginal flooding alone had little or no detectable effect on outcome, whereas exposure to the phobic situation had a consistent positive effect. It was concluded that imaginal flooding was useless unless the patients had the opportunity to practice *(in vivo)* what they had experienced in imagination after returning home from the session. *In vivo* and imaginal flooding differed in effectiveness in directly reducing fears but were equal in facilitating practice between sessions. However, *in vivo* practice appeared to be the main determinant of outcome. Johnston *et al.* concluded that imaginal flooding is useful only when combined with live practice, and as a means of facilitating that practice, but that, in and of itself, has little effect.

In a study of obsessive-compulsive neurotics, Rabavilas, Boulougouris, and Stephanis (1976) used a Latin-square crossover design to compare the effects of flooding *in vivo* versus flooding in fantasy across 2 levels of duration of exposure (short and long). All sessions were 2 hr in length and each condition (duration of exposure × mode of exposure) was offered to the patient for 2 sessions over 1 week. Thus, all patients received all 4 conditions in 8 sessions over a 4-week period. The order in which treatments were given was counterbalanced. All treatment sessions consisted of a total of 80 min of exposure time during each 2-hr treatment session. In the long-exposure condition, the full 80 min of exposure was offered all at once, regardless of whether treatment was *in vivo* or in fantasy. During the short-exposure condition, the patient was exposed to bursts of 10-min segments interspersed with 5 min of "neutral imagery or talk." Rabavilas *et al.* concluded that *in vivo* flooding was "far superior" to fantasy flooding regardless of the duration of exposure.

It is clear that for phobias and for obsessive-compulsive disorders *in vivo* flooding is superior to imaginal or fantasy flooding when evaluated immediately following therapy. However, all of the above studies used experimental designs that do not allow for follow-up. It could be that the long-term effect of imaginal flooding might enhance *in vivo* exposure. To test this notion, Foa, Steketee, Turner, and Fischer (1980) compared two groups of obsessive-compulsives. One group was treated with imaginal exposure and *in vivo* exposure, while the other was given only *in vivo* exposure. Foa *et al.* found that, while the group treated only with *in vivo* exposure initially fared as well as the group treated with both imaginal and *in vivo* exposure, an 11-month follow-up revealed that patients in the *in vivo* only group relapsed at a significantly higher rate.

In a recent study of agoraphobics, Chambless, Foa, Groves, and

Goldstein (1980) also found that at a 4-month follow-up imaginal exposure was just as effective as *in vivo* exposure in controlling at least two types of anxiety symptoms—avoidance behavior and self-report of fear. Yet, *in vivo* exposure did appear to be more effective for two other outcome measures (anxious mood and panic). Chambless *et al.* concluded that "We may be abandoning imaginal exposure too precipitously."

From a learning theory standpoint, we agree with Chambless *et al.*, but add that fantasy or *in vivo* exposure is most effective depending on whether real or fantasy stimuli were most prominent during fear conditioning. Where a concrete external set of stimuli are the primary fear stimuli (e.g., phobias), *in vivo* exposure to these stimuli should yield a more rapid extinction than fantasy exposure to the same set of stimuli. This follows from the fact that the fantasy stimuli would be further removed on the generalization of extinction gradient than the *in vivo* stimuli. However, in complex neurotic disorders, thoughts and images may have formed part of the stimulus complex during the original fear-conditioning events. In such cases, presentation of these internal stimuli in imagery would be indicated. Further, from a practical standpoint, many complex fear cues are not easily presented *in vivo*. As mentioned earlier, a client who fears disease or death cannot be exposed to the necessary fantasies repeatedly *in vivo*. Similarly, obsessional thoughts not accompanied by specific compulsive behavior, or anxieties stimulated by unpleasant memories, are not easily treated without the use of imaginal exposure. Finally, even if the therapist is using a simple *in vivo* flooding technique, imaginal exposure can be used to prepare or instruct the client in how to carry out *in vivo* flooding on his or her own.

Optimal Length of Exposure Session

Several studies have attempted to determine whether exposure should be presented in lengthy or brief segments. Research at the human analogue level (see Chapter 2) proved lengthy (massed) exposures more effective than many brief (spaced) exposures. At the animal level, however, there was no difference between massed and spaced exposure.

The first study to attempt to evalute this at the clinical level was carried out by Stern and Marks (1973), who treated 16 agoraphobics in a Latin-square design with 4 sessions of long or short flooding, both in fantasy and in practice. Each client participated in every treatment condition, and all clients were given four 2-hr sessions of tape-recorded flooding in imagination followed by 2 hr of flooding *in vivo*. Thus, all subjects received the same total amount of flooding. During half of the sessions, imaginal flooding was given in "bursts" of 10-min segments for a total of 2 hr of exposure time. For the other half of the sessions, long imaginal flooding involved 80 min of continuous flooding scenes followed by 40 continuous min of neutral scenes. In the *in vivo* practice sessions, short flooding consisted of four 30-min periods of exposure separated by 30 min of rest, whereas in the long flooding, all subjects received 2 hr of continuous *in vivo* practice. Physiological and behavioral measures, psychological tests, and ratings by "assessors" found no significant difference between long and short fantasy sessions. Both were ineffective. *In vivo* flooding resulted in improvement, regardless of session length, although long flooding *in vivo* was significantly more effective than the four 30 min *in vivo* periods. No follow-up was attempted. In a similar study already discussed, Rabavilas *et al.* (1976) found that for obsessive-compulsive disorders prolonged flooding was superior to shorter exposure.

Based on these two studies then, it would appear that sessions of long duration (even up to 3 hr) are more effective than shorter sessions for *in vivo* flooding. This is true even if the total time of exposure over all sessions remains constant for both conditions. Nevertheless, exposure was effective in reducing avoidance behavior, regardless of session length. Thus, even though sessions of long duration are preferred, exposure is still a viable treatment technique for the practicing clinician whose session length is often determined by more practical considerations.

Homework Exposure

Stampfl and Levis (1969) suggest that implosive-therapy clients be given homework assignments that involve rehearsing implosive scenes on their own between therapy sessions. This appears to be a reasonable adjunct to therapy. Exposure is effective in reducing anxiety and the more of it the better. Few studies, however, have directly tested this hypothesis. One study that did not include a control group found that for agoraphobics exposure treatment *in vivo* was effective when carried out at home with only very minimal therapist involvement (Mathews, Teasdale, Munby, Johnston, & Shaw, 1977). Similarly, Emmelkamp and Ultee (1974) found that their "self-observation" treatment procedure, which also involves minimal therapist contact, was just as effective as an exposure procedure which used intensive therapist contact. Emmelkamp (1974) replicated these results. Griest, Marks, Berlin, Gournay, and Noshirvani (1980) also successfully treated a mixed sample of phobics and obsessive-compulsives with homework assignment only. All of these studies involved *in vivo* exposure. We know of no study that specifically tested the effects of imaginal homework.

We routinely give both *in vivo* and imaginal homework assignments to our clients. We find that self-exposure is an economical treatment and that homework assignments have "face validity." After all, the *goal* of therapy is to have clients expose themselves to the fear cues *on their own*. Yet, from the clinician's viewpoint, the extent to which homework is assigned should depend on clinical considerations (e.g., client's ego strength, motivation, and support of significant others). These considerations are discussed in more detail in Chapters 4 and 5.

Group versus Individual Treatment

Many studies (e.g., Chambless & Goldstein, 1981; Hand, Lamontagne & Marks, 1974; Teasdale *et al.*, 1977) of both *in vivo* and imaginal flooding have found group exposure treatment to be effective. Two studies directly compared individual versus group treatment. Hafner and Marks (1976), using *in vivo* flooding, found that group treatment was somewhat better than individual treatment. Butollo and Mittalstaedt (1977) found that individual treatment was more effective. Differences in these results may be due to the fact that Hafner and Marks used agoraphobics while Butollo and Mittelstaedt treated a variety of specific phobics.

The financial advantage and time economy of group treatment are obvious. On the other hand, many clinicians do not see enough clients with the same disorder to assemble a group. The scant evidence to date would support either individual or group exposure as effective treatments for at least some anxiety disorders.

The Effect of Group Cohesiveness on Exposure

Hand, Lamontagne, and Marks (1974) hypothesized that social cohesion in the group would affect patient motivation and anxiety in the phobic situation. In this study 25 agoraphobics were randomly assigned to 6 therapy groups (4 to 5 subjects in each). Three of these groups were structured to foster group cohesion, and the other 3 groups were unstructured to minimize cohesion. The structured group met in a traditional group-therapy format before and after experiencing *in vivo* flooding. These subjects were encouraged to interact and to discuss their problems with one another. In the unstructured groups, members were given little opportunity to interact and were told to stay clear of "significant" topics when they did talk to one another. All patients received 3

4-hr treatments over a 1-week period. Behavioral tests and rating scales completed by both clients and "assessors" indicated that overall outcome for all groups was at least as good as reported in previous trials with individual patients. Immediately following therapy, patients in all groups improved significantly with no differences between groups. However, at 3- and 6-month follow-ups, clients in structured groups showed greater improvement and had fewer relapses and dropouts than members of the unstructured groups. Hand *et al.* suggested that posttreatment interaction between members of the structured groups helped them to maintain their gains.

Teasdale, Walsh, Lancashire, and Mathews (1977) attempted to replicate this study. In their study, improvement also occurred in both structured and unstructured groups but did not continue in either group during follow-up. Teasdale *et al.* concluded that, regardless of the cohesiveness of the group, further improvement at follow-up depends on whether subjects continue to expose themselves to feared cues.

It would seem reasonable that individuals treated with exposure in groups would fare better in member support resulted in continued exposure to feared situations. The fostering support geared toward such continued exposure makes good clinical sense.

Client Response during Treatment

Based on two-factor theory, Stampfl and Levis have always maintained that to be effective, the therapist must elicit anxiety during implosive sessions so as to allow for subsequent extinction of the conditioned emotional response. Evidence from clinical samples supporting this notion is not strong. A number of studies that did not directly vary this factor have reported no correlation between arousal level during treatment and outcome (e.g., Boudewyns & Wilson, 1972; Stern & Marks, 1973; Watson & Marks, 1971).

Several studies have attempted to manipulate the anxiety response of subjects as an independent variable (through the use of tranquilizers or relaxation training) such that the anxiety level of one group was significantly greater than a comparison group in response to the same flooding scenes (Chambless, Foa, Groves, & Goldstein, 1979; Gelder, Bancroft, Gath, Johnston, Mathews, & Shaw, 1973; Hafner & Marks, 1976; Mathews, Johnston, Shaw, & Gelder, 1974). In all but the Chambless study, the results of these trials found no evidence that high arousal during exposure increased effectiveness of the therapy. Chambless *et al.* used imaginal flooding and found that high anxiety during flooding enhanced short-term treatment effects for agoraphobics. However, a follow-up to that study could not confirm this result 16 weeks following treatment.

There appears to be little empirical support for the notion that eliciting high anxiety is a necessary condition for effective exposure treatment. On the other hand, many of the above studies "proved" that the client's response during treatment is not related to outcome by accepting the null hypothesis of no significant difference between groups. This type of backward experimental result leaves many questions. For example, it could be that there is an optimal level of anxiety associated with positive outcome (Foa & Chambless, 1978) and that both the comparison groups in these studies fell within that range. As also noted by Foa and Chambless, anxiety may appear in many response modes (subjective or verbal report, behavioral and/or physiological) and these generally do not correlate highly at any point. All of the above studies used rough estimates of anxiety, often measured only by self-report.

From a clinical standpoint, the eliciting of anxiety during exposure sessions has at least practical value. As will be noted in Chapter 4, observing anxiety in the client is probably the best indication that the material presented is meaningful. Also, repeatedly presenting anxiety-eliciting material to the point where the client ultimately experiences a reduction in arousal increases the credibility of the treatment.

Psychotropic Medications with Exposure

As previously reviewed, analogue studies have not shown any consistent advantage for administering exposure under drugged conditions. At the clinical level, several investigators have examined the effects of the use of psychotropic medication during exposure to enhance the effect of treatment. Johnston and Gath (1973) compared the effects of 20 mg of diazepam with that of a placebo, administered under otherwise similar conditions, during *in vivo* exposure with agoraphobics. They concluded that exposure was more effective when given in conjunction with the active medication. Unfortunately, the study is markedly flawed by the fact that only four subjects made up the sample. Consequently, the parametric inferential statistic used by these investigators is of doubtful validity.

In a more substantial trial of the effects of diazepam, Marks, Viswanathan, Lipsedge, and Gardner (1972) used a crossover design to expose 18 specific phobics for 2 hr to the "real phobic situation" under 2 conditions: (1) either 4 hr after ingestion of an oral elixir of diazepam

(0.1 diazepam per kilogram of bodyweight) or (2) at "peak" effect, 1 hr after ingestion of diazepam. All subjects taking the placebo elixir were exposed in the same manner as the subjects who had taken the diazepam. Each subject received 36 treatment sessions. Treatments were counterbalanced for order effects. All treatment conditions resulted in significant positive effects on most measures, but in general the peak group treatment was not as effective as the 4-hr group. Both active treatment groups were more effective than the placebo group. Marks *et al.* concluded that phobics might be best treated if they are given sedation approximately 4 hr before the exposure *in vivo.* Again, the crossover design did not allow for follow-up.

In a similar study that did allow for follow-up, Hafner and Marks (1976) found that exposure *in vivo* carried out 3 to 4 hr after administration of diazepam was more effective than treatment offered ½ hr after diazepam ingestion, although this advantage disappeared at the 3 and 6-month follow-up.

One study evaluated the effects of an intravenous sedative given during exposure. Hussain (1971) combined intravenous thiopental and exposure in the treatment of agoraphobics ($n = 40$). Twenty patients were treated with either six 45-min sessions of imaginal flooding, assisted by 20 cc of 1.25% solution of thiopental (infused slowly intravenously) followed by the same number of sessions, assisted by 20 cc intravenous saline infusion, or vice versa. The other 20 subjects were treated with the same number of sessions of systematic desensitization, assisted in the same fashion with either the active drug or the saline. Results found that thiopental facilitated flooding, but was not effective for desensitization. Again, it is unfortunate that the crossover design in the study disallowed evaluation of the effects at follow-up.

One psychotropic medication that appears to be effective with agoraphobics treated with exposure is imipramine (Chambless & Goldstein, 1981; Zitrin, 1981; Zitrin, Klein, & Woerner, 1980; Zitrin, Klein, Lindenman, Tobak, Rock, Kaplan, & Ganz, 1976). However, no study to date has systematically varied imipramine administration and exposure treatment in a manner that would determine the long-term interactive effects of these two treatments. In one study Zitrin *et al.* (1980) found that imipramine did enhance the effect of a relatively graded *in vivo* exposure when compared to a placebo drug. In this study 76 female phobics were treated with *in vivo* exposure and either imipramine or placebo medications. Most outcome measures immediately following therapy and at the 3-month follow-up favored the imipramine-treated group. However, all patients continued to improve at the same rate following therapy. A longer follow-up might have eventually found no difference between the two groups after the imipramine-treated group reached a plateau. Further, since subjects continued to receive either saline or imipramine throughout follow-up, it is impossible to determine the extent of any relapse after imipramine administration had been discontinued.

In general, if there are positive effects of imipramine with agoraphobics, they probably occur because (1) the drug is effective in reducing panic attacks and (2) exposure-treated patients who are also treated with imipramine are less likely to drop out of therapy (Chambless & Goldstein, 1981). There is little evidence that the drug is helpful for specific phobic behavior.

Based on rather meager evidence, it might be suggested that psychotropic medication may increase the effectiveness of exposure (both *in vivo* and imaginal) under certain conditions, yet the long-term effectiveness of drug-assisted exposure is unknown.

Graded versus Nongraded Exposure

Several studies already reviewed have compared the effects of systematic desensitization with flooding. In a sense, these studies address the relative effects of graded versus nongraded exposure. However, desensitization treatment usually involves some form of relaxation training and exposure, which depends on the client's emotional response, is extremely gradual. Several studies are reviewed below that compared graded versus nongraded flooding, although avoiding the confounding variable of deep muscle relaxation.

Everaerd, Rijken, and Emmelkamp (1973) used a crossover design to investigate the effects of flooding, both in imagination and *in vivo*, as compared to the relatively more graded procedure that they described as "successive approximations." In the latter procedure, 14 subjects were instructed to "go into the street and stay outside until you begin to feel uncomfortable or tense." They were further instructed to return when they felt uncomfortable. Sessions lasted 90 min. In the flooding sessions, 45 min of flooding in imagination was immediately followed by 45 min of *in vivo* flooding. Clients were required to remain in the phobic situation for the duration of the session. All subjects participated in both types of exposure in a manner that counterbalanced for order effects. No non-treated or placebo control group was included in the study. Assessments were made (1) prior to treatment, (2) at crossover, (3) following treatment, and (4) at 3-month follow-up. Based on self-reports, psychological test data, physiological response, and *in vivo* behavioral tests, subjects in both exposure conditions improved on most measures with no significant differences between the groups. Both groups at follow-up had significantly increased the amount of time spent in the phobic situation and had significantly decreased scores related to phobic anxiety.

Boersma, den Hengst, Dekker, and Emmelkamp (1976) used a 2 × 2 factorial design to compare the effects of gradual treatment (graded exposure) to nongraded exposure, and modeling to no modeling. Thirteen obsessive-compulsive clients were treated using a crossover design which resulted in small unequal sample sizes for each cell (four, three, two, and four). The flooding condition consisted of a total response–prevention procedure. In this condition, subjects were required to remain in the most aversive stimulus situation they could think of (e.g., continually contaminated hands) and were not allowed to make a ritualistic response (such as handwashing) throughout the entire treatment session. In the graded-exposure condition, a form of gradual response prevention was used. All items in the hierarchy were practiced starting with the easiest (e.g., touching the outside of a wastebasket with one finger) to the most difficult (e.g., both hands in the toilet). In the modeling groups, the two conditions were used but initially the therapist modeled the behavior for the client. All clients were given four pretest sessions followed by 15 treatment sessions. Two follow-up sessions were held one month and three months following the last treatment session. Outcome was evaluated using *in vivo* behavioral ratings, therapist ratings, and various physiological scales for both symptom-specific and more general personality and emotional factors. There were no significant differences between the groups. In fact, only two of the 22 measures used showed significant differences at the .05 level. All groups showed highly significant pre- to posttreatment changes which were not depleted at follow-up. In a later study, Emmelkamp and Kraanen (1977) also found that a more graded exposure plus response prevention was effective with obsessive-compulsives, but the technique was not compared to nongraded exposure.

The results of these studies indicate that grading is not a particularly important factor in flooding. However, it has been shown that the amount of exposure time is significant. Thus, to the extent that it reduces the amount of exposure time, a graded approach is less efficient than a more direct exposure. On the other hand, it is often difficult to contract with the client to use a totally nongraded approach. In the clinic the degree of grading is often determined by negotiation with the client.

Treating Obsessive Thoughts Unaccompanied by Compulsion

Patients who suffer from obsessions often engage in compulsive rituals that serve to reduce the anxiety caused by the obsessional thoughts. Therapeutic exposure for these patients may simply involve not allowing them to engage in the compulsive ritual. Flooding occurs when the patient can no longer make the avoidance response (compulsive ritual). However, in our clinical experience, the obsessional patients that do not engage in compulsive rituals are more difficult to treat than those patients that do engage in ritual behavior.

To research this issue, Stern (1978) treated nonritualizing obsessive patients with a variety of techniques, including thought stopping, relaxation therapy, and "satiation," a technique virtually indistinguishable from implosive therapy or imaginal flooding. Also all patients were given a course of amitriptyline. The conditions of treatment were so confounded (triple crossover design) that it is difficult to determine whether anything was effective. In general, the author concluded that the overall results were poor, regardless of the techniques used, although the flooding manipulation appeared to be effective with at least one type of obsessive thought (e.g., "horror–disgust ruminations"). This study is in contrast with an earlier study by Emmelkamp and Kwee (1977) in which exposure in imagination was compared to thought stopping. In that study both techniques were mildly effective in reducing obsessive thoughts but there was no difference in effectiveness between the two.

Direct Exposure versus Other Psychotherapeutic Techniques in Treating Anxiety Disorders

Several studies have compared the effects of direct exposure with systematic desensitization. In the first study Boulougouris, Marks, and Marset (1971) found that flooding was significantly superior to desensitization for agoraphobia, although both flooding and systematic desensitization were comparable for specific phobias. The study used a crossover design and it was therefore impossible to determine whether these effects were maintained at follow-up.

In a more complex study that did allow for follow-up, Gelder *et al.* (1973) compared flooding with systematic desensitization and a control treatment. Flooding consisted of a combination of both *in vivo* and imaginal exposure. Immediately following therapy, both the flooding and systematic desensitization groups showed significant improvement over the control procedure for most outcome measures. Gelder *et al.* reported that, although the differences were not always significant between systematic desensitization and the flooding group, for most variables flooding was found to be superior. At 6-month follow-up, however, attrition appeared to reduce differences between the groups to nonsignificance.

In a third study, Crowe, Marks, Agras, and Leitenberg (1972) used a crossover design to compare the effects of systematic desensitization, implosive therapy, and shaping or "reinforced practice" with 14 phobic patients. Four patients were agoraphobics and 10 suffered from specific phobias. Both systematic desensitization and implosive therapy were carried out in imagination. The shaping procedure was essentially a graded *in vivo* exposure with verbal rewards offered to clients who performed well. In this condition, patients were instructed to approach as close to the feared object or situation as possible but to retreat before they became unduly anxious. The therapist's praise was given when patients "exceeded a criterion" and the criterion was raised "in accordance with improving performance." All patients received treatments in random order. Each of the three treatments was administered over 50-min sessions (12 sessions in all). Results indicated that, on behavioral tests of approach to the feared cue, the *in vivo* shaping technique was the most effective. The more generalized symptoms of depression, anxiety, panic, and depersonalization as rated by both the patient and significant others were not affected by any of the techniques. The order, in terms of effectiveness, for the three treatment conditions suggested that *in vivo* shaping was more effective than implosion, which in turn was more effective than systematic desensitization. This same order was more consistent across measures for the four agoraphobic patients. It was concluded that when agoraphobic and phobic patients are treated with exposure techniques, a graded *in vivo* exposure is superior to either imaginal flooding or systematic desensitization. An interesting result of this study was that patients preferred to be treated with desensitization even though graded shaping was the most effective procedure. Again, the crossover design does not allow for any follow-up and, therefore, this conclusion must remain tentative.

As already reported, Hussain (1971) found imaginal flooding superior to systematic desensitization in treating agoraphobics, but the results were confounded by the fact that during therapy patients received intravenous injections of either an active drug or placebo.

One study (Emmelkamp, Kuipers, & Eggeraat, 1978) compared the effectiveness of five 2-hr group sessions of either prolonged exposure *in vivo* or cognitive restructuring. In the latter type of treatment, anxious subjects were trained to abandon anxiety-inducing cognitions and to voice more productive self-statements. Twenty agoraphobics received both treatments in a crossover design. At posttest, combined results showed improvements on all variables. However, for most outcome measures, exposure was superior to cognitive restructuring and on none of the outcome measures was the reverse true.

Several studies have compared the effects of flooding *in vivo* with modeling and/or a combination of the two. In a series of three small studies, Rachman, Hodgson, and Marks (1971), Hodgson, Rachman, and Marks (1972) and Rachman, Marks, and Hodgson (1973) treated a total of 20 severe obsessive-compulsive patients with a combination of *in vivo* flooding and modeling. Although these studies all contained small samples and used crossover designs, the fact that the results were replicated makes the three taken together a significant contribution. In all three studies, flooding plus modeling was found to be significantly more effective than a relaxation treatment alone. In another study with a small sample size, Boersma *et al.* (1976) found that modeling did not augment the effects of either graded or nongraded exposure when treating obsessive-compulsive disorders. This study is suspect, however, in that the number of subjects per cell was so small that the inferential parametric statistic used to evaluate the difference between the groups may have been unreliable.

One controlled outcome study (Shaw 1979) tested the effects of flooding with social phobics. This study compared desensitization to imaginal flooding and a form of social skills training. Thirty social phobics were divided into three groups, each of which was treated with one of the above techniques. Measures were taken pre- and posttreatment and at 6-month follow-up. Assessment was carried out by a "blind" rater. A behavioral test was also used in which the patient was asked to "attempt the highest possible item on the hierarchy and rate it on a 0 to 10 scale of anxiety before and after treatment and at 6 months following treatment." Results found that all three treatments were effective for most outcome measures, including those reported by the rater, the patient's own ratings, and the behavioral tests. It was concluded that since all treatments were effective, the decision of which to use should be made on the basis of either cost or patient acceptability. Shaw conjectured that because flooding is "clearly" low on patient acceptability and social skills training is very costly, desensitization is, therefore, the treatment of choice. In our own experience, however, flooding is usually a more economical treatment technique, taking less time than desensitization. Shaw's study has other inherent problems. For instance, time was held constant. Perhaps if ratings had been taken midway through treatment, differences between the groups may have been evident. Another problem with the study was that the therapists were not of equal experience and the experience factor was further confounded with the conditions of treatment. It was reported that the seven therapists providing the flooding and desensitization treatment consisted of four psychiatrists, two psychologists, and one senior clinical student;

experience with behavior therapy varied considerably among the therapists. Social skills training, however, was carried out by two therapists, both of whom had considerable experience in this form of treatment.

Turner, Hersen, Bellack, and Wells (1978) investigated the effects of imaginal flooding versus response prevention using a single-case time series design with each of the two subjects. Turner *et al.* concluded that response prevention was effective in reducing ritualistic behavior, although the effects of flooding added little to the outcome. However, in our reading of the graphs offered by these authors, the results of this study do not appear to support this conclusion. In fact, for one subject, the intervention of a flooding procedure to the response–prevention technique actually decreased ritualistic behavior during the baseline period more than during a baseline period that followed response prevention alone. In the second case, flooding was added to a response–prevention manipulation after a total of 37 days of response–prevention therapy. This did not reduce the ritualistic behaviors anymore than what had resulted from the response–prevention intervention alone. However, as the authors themselves note, almost every ritualistic behavior evaluated was already occurring at close to zero rate. Further reduction was difficult, if not impossible. There were at least two other problems: (1) the total time (days) that each subject received response prevention was much greater than the number of days they received flooding and (2) the two techniques were never counterbalanced for order effect; response prevention was always offered first. In sum, we would agree with Turner *et al.* that response prevention appeared effective in reducing rituals, but nothing can be said about the effects of imaginal flooding one way or the other.

In the study by Griest *et al.* (1980) reported earlier, the obvious was finally tested. These authors compared the effects of exposure versus an "avoidance manipulation" on 13 phobic and 4 obsessive ritualizing patients. In the exposure condition, one half of the patients were instructed to do homework which consisted of "confronting" stimuli that evoked fear, for as long as possible. The other half were instructed to avoid consistently any and all contact with the stimuli that evoked fear. Griest *et al.* reported that changes after each treatment were small but consistent and that phobics improved with exposure instructions significantly more than with avoidance instructions. Avoidance resulted in a slight increase in phobic behavior and anxiety for both phobics and compulsive ritualizers. The major problem with this study was that the investigators used a crossover design. One addition to the study that gave it more creditibility, however, was the use of an expectancy check in which "care was taken" to introduce expectation for change in the two conditions. Griest *et al.* found that there were no differences in expectancies prior to treatment but, after treatment, the exposure-condition subjects had greater expectancy for positive change than did the avoidance group.

Exposure Techniques Used with Other Disorders

If we assume that almost any psychological disorder has an anxiety component, then exposure techniques should be applicable to a variety of disorders. In this section, studies are reviewed that evaluate the effects of exposure with several different types of disorders. In some cases, these studies include a heterogeneous sample of patients.

Psychiatric Inpatients and Outpatients

The first controlled study of implosive therapy was carried out by Hogan (1966). In this trial, 50 psychotic inpatients participated as subjects. Twenty-four were given "traditional treatment" and 26 were "assigned to implosive therapists." The two groups were matched on various demographic and social variables. Neither the therapists nor the patients were aware that they were participating in a study. Pre- and posttreatment MMPI (Minnesota Multiphasic Personality Inventory) scores and posttherapy discharge rates were evaluated one year following hospitalization. Assessment of MMPI scale scores indicated that significant downward shifts occurred more often in the implosive-therapy group than in the control group. Furthermore, one year following hospitalization, significantly more patients in the implosive group had been discharged from the hospital.

In a more comprehensive design, Boudewyns and Wilson (1972) studied three groups (n = 12 each) of VA psychiatric inpatients. One group received implosive therapy and a second received a nonstructured form of desensitization described by Wilson and Smith (1968). Subjects in both of these active treatment groups also received the usual hospital milieu treatment. The third group of patients, who served as controls, received only the milieu treatment. Although subjects were limited to patients who had peaks on either scale 2 (Depression) or 7 (Psychasthenia) on the pretreatment MMPIs, all groups were diagnostically heterogeneous. Before treatment, after treatment, and at the 6-month follow-up, both the MMPI and the Mooney Problem Checklist were administered and progress toward individualized goals was rated by the patient and a significant other. Employment and hospitalization status were also recorded during the year following treatment. Both treatment groups improved significantly over the control group. The implosive group, however, improved on more measures and maintained improvement better at the 6-month follow-up.

At one and five years following treatment, rehospitalization and the employment histories of the subjects were again evaluated (Boudewyns, 1975; Boudewyns & Wilson, 1972). At 1-year follow-up, rehospitalization rates were low for all groups, and there were no significant differences between the groups in the months spent in gainful employment. At 5-year follow-up, the implosive-therapy group had significantly lower rehospitalization rates than the milieu group. Although the hospital milieu had been active, expensive, and offered a variety of therapeutic activities, the control group, which received only the milieu treatment, appeared to benefit minimally, if at all, from treatment (Boudewyns, 1974).

In a third study, Lev' and Carrera (1967) conducted a well-controlled study of implosive therapy with psychiatric outpatients. Forty clients were assigned to receive either implosive therapy or one of three control treatments. One control group received insight and supportive therapy; the second was given "conventional" therapy; and the third consisted of a nontreated waiting list control. Therapy was limited to 10 sessions. On the MMPI that was administered to all subjects prior to and following treatment, only the implosive-therapy group showed a consistent shift away from psychopathology. The study can be criticized on the basis that the outcome was based entirely on the MMPI scale score changes and no behavioral data or follow-ups were offered.

The above three studies obtained positive effects using only imaginal exposure. This becomes noteworthy, given the controversy regarding the relative effects of *in vivo* versus imaginal flooding. The primary weakness of the above studies is that they all used a heterogeneous patient sample. On the other hand, it would seem reasonable to assume that all psychiatric patients have problems with anxiety management and that any therapy technique which effectively reduces anxiety should be helpful. Also, using more heterogeneous patients makes it possible to acquire larger samples. Finally, two of the studies had long follow-ups of a year or more. Taken together, these three studies are strong support for the effectiveness of implosive therapy or flooding in imagination for a broad range of psychiatric patients.

Agitated Depression

Hannie and Adams (1974) hypothesized that, because anxiety is a significant component of agitated depression, flooding should be an effective technique for treating this disorder. In this study, 27 female inpatients with symptoms of anxiety and depression were randomly divided into 3 treatment groups. All subjects received the usual ward milieu therapy; 2 of the 3 groups also received either supportive therapy (nondirective) or imaginal flooding for a maximum of 9 sessions or until discharge.

Outcome measures included pre- to postassessment scores on the Mental Status Schedule (MSS), the Multiple Affect Adjective Checklist (MAACL), the Fear Survey Schedule (FSS), and the Digit Symbol Subtest of the WAIS. On the MSS and MAACL, flooding was found to be the most effective treatment technique. The study did not include a formal follow-up.

One interesting result of this study was that compared to the controls, subjects in the flooding group used more medication in the first half of the study and less in the last half. Hannie and Adams interpret this as support for the extinction theory of flooding.

Alcoholism

Newton and Stein (1974) assessed the effects of implosive therapy with alcoholics. In this study, all patients were detoxified and received milieu treatment for 25 days during hospitalization. Milieu treatment included group therapy, behavior modification, family therapy, Alcoholics Anonymous activities, and education groups. A control group of 29 patients received no further treatment. In addition to the milieu treatment, 16 patients were also given implosive therapy, while another 16 received "brief psychotherapy." Outcome measures included various personality measures (Gough's Adjective Checklist and the Standard Situation Test) and rating scales of improvement that were completed by staff and ward personnel. All three groups improved, but there was no significant difference among them. In other words, neither implosive therapy nor brief psychotherapy brought about improvement in functioning over and above the results of the milieu treatment. Follow-up was conducted at 1, 3, 6, 9, and 12 months, but these data were not reported.

Based on this one study, it would appear that implosive therapy is not a particularly effective treatment for alcoholic clients who are receiving other forms of treatment at the same time. It may be that those alcoholics who drink primarily to reduce anxiety would be helped by implosive therapy, however, Newton and Stein did not relate anxiety level to outcome.

Emotionally Disturbed Retardates

Silvestri (1977) argued that because implosive therapy "deemphasizes the importance of insight and problem-solving ability," the therapy technique may be especially useful with emotionally disturbed retardates. Twenty-four emotionally disturbed retarded adults and adolescents, matched for age, sex, race, and IQ, were randomly assigned to one treatment and two control groups. Patients in the treatment group received 10 sessions of implosive therapy. Patients in one control group received no active treatment other than the milieu activities offered to all patients. Those in the second control group were given 10 sessions of "pseudo treatment oriented discussion." Using a variety of behavioral, subjective, and clinical ratings, Silvestri found that the implosive-therapy group showed significantly greater improvement on all measures than the two control groups. At a 6-week follow-up, the subjects in the implosive-therapy group had maintained their gains.

Heroin Addiction

Hirt and Greenfield (1979) examined the effectiveness of implosive therapy with heroin addicts during detoxification from methadone. In this interesting study, 16 addicts were treated with either implosive therapy or eclectic counseling. Eight subjects in a third group were not treated and were used as controls. The results indicated that implosive therapy was effective in reducing the subject's requests for methadone during detoxification. There was no difference between the eclectic group and the nontreated controls in terms of the amount of methadone used during detoxification. The authors concluded:

> Based on Mowrer's two-factor theory, pathological behavior develops when previously neutral stimuli become paired with painful or aversive ones and come to serve as cues for recurrence of the aversive situation. These classically conditioned cues acquire sufficient anxiety-producing properties that their occurrence, per se, is an aversive event. Responses that terminate or otherwise circumvent their occurrence served both to motivate and to reinforce (by anxiety reduction) the pathological behavior. Applied to the methadone patient, previous withdrawal experience represents the classical conditioning and the slight semantic changes serve as cues to motivate the maladaptive behavior. (p. 982–983)

They suggest that implosive therapy serves to extinguish the anxiety associated with these cues, and, subsequently, the ingestion of drugs—the avoidance response.

Insomnia

In a rather unusual application of the technique, Carrera and Elenewski (1980) used implosive therapy to treat 200 insomniacs. It is difficult to determine whether this should be considered an analogue study or a clinical level study. The problem treated was of clinical significance but the clients were volunteer psychology students from an introductory psychology class.

Carrera and Elenewski had four therapy conditions: (1) death implosion, (2) general implosion, (3) ocean tape, and (4) wait-list control. In the death implosion condition, clients were asked to

> visualize lying in bed at home and having difficulty in falling asleep. They were then asked to attend to various bodily sensations and progressively become involved in the fantasy of having a strange disease. After considerable concern, rumination, and progressive physical and emotional difficulty, they were instructed to fantasize their own death.

In condition two, general implosion, clients were asked to fantasize scenes "centered around a gradual loss of self control, acting out various socially forbidden behaviors and eventually becoming psychotic." In condition three, subjects were told to "imagine themselves on a beach and then to allow their fantasies to go wherever they wished." They listened to a tape which was "composed of recordings of the ocean taken at various locations and especially intermixed with a computer system." (p. 733). Results indicated that only the death implosion condition was significantly more effective than the wait-list control. There were no differences between any of the other conditions.

Summary

Nongraded exposure techniques are clinically effective treatments for several anxiety disorders, particularly phobias and obsessive-compulsive disorders. It also appears that flooding *in vivo* is more effective than flooding in imagination, at least for agoraphobics. However, both techniques are effective and imaginal flooding does augment the effects of *in vivo* flooding, especially at follow-up. There is some indication that *in vivo* flooding in the milieu of a group will help agoraphobics maintain and even continue their gains and prevent relapse after the final treatment if group members are allowed to interact and support one another. Group support may exert its positive influence by encouraging continued exposure to fear cues. It has also been found that prolonged exposure of up to three hours per session may be more effective than exposure of a shorter duration, even if the total treatment time is held constant.

Research with drugs has found that diazepam, given 3 to 4 hours prior to treatment, may augment the effects of flooding in imagination combined with *in vivo* experience. Imipramine may augment the effects of exposure treatment for agoraphobics who suffer panic attacks and may also serve to keep agoraphobics in therapy longer, thus increasing exposure time.

Although the evidence for the effectiveness of exposure techniques overwhelmingly favors their use with anxiety-based disorders, some issues still need to be explored. For instance, more evidence is needed to support the long-term effects of treatment. Most of the studies reviewed used crossover designs that make it impossible to carry out a meaningful follow-up. In those studies that did not use crossover designs, patients were followed for a relatively short time after therapy (usually not more than three to six months). However, data from several studies support the long-term positive effects (one to five years) of formalized implosive therapy applied to a heterogeneous sample of psychiatric inpatients and outpatients.

Other disorders for which there is at least some evidence that therapeutic exposure may be effective include emotional disturbance in retardants, agitated depression, and insomnia. One study of the effects of implosive therapy with alcoholics found no evidence that this exposure technique added to the effects of an active milieu therapy. However, another study found that implosive techniques may aid in the withdrawal from heroin addiction.

Compared to graded exposure, nongraded exposure is more time efficient and was usually found to be more effective, but for specific phobias, grading may make little difference. Finally, nowhere in the clinical outcome literature is there any evidence that therapeutic exposure is harmful to clients, even to clients with low ego strength.

Case Reports

Case studies are of little significance in determining the effectiveness of a treatment with the possible exception of single-case time-series designs. They tend not to confirm or to refute effectiveness. They do, however, exemplify various techniques that are used to rectify types of problem behaviors. Furthermore, case studies may be useful in suggesting possible procedures that can be attempted when other, more traditional treatment regimens have been ineffective.

In this section, we have selected for review several published case studies that demonstrate the application of therapeutic exposure to either difficult or unusual problems and/or disorders.

Adult Phobias with Obsessive-Compulsive Features

Eye Patch Phobia. Thomas and Rapp (1977) reported a study of a 40-year-old female suffering from an "eye patch phobia." The client became anxious when seeing a person or a picture of a person wearing an eye patch; even the word "patch" generated anxiety. Her fears had generalized to the point where she would not venture from her house and where she worried incessantly that a family member would injure his or her eye and need to use an eye patch. Nineteen weekly sessions of aversion relief did not improve her condition, so a continuous 9-hr flooding procedure was instituted. Measurements of physiological, behavioral, and subjective responses to imagined and live stimulation were made one week prior to and one and two weeks following the flooding session. Improvement occurred in the behavioral measure with no deterioration at the second follow-up. Physiological and subjective measures showed less improvement, but these modest improvements were generally maintained at the 2-week follow-up.

Germ and Crowd Phobia. Rubadeau and Rubadeau (1972) treated a female undergraduate who had suffered from a germ and crowd phobia for six years. Although the phobia had become so severe that it disabled the client in any social situation, it was completely alleviated after 12 30-min sessions of implosive therapy. The phobia had not recurred at the 16-month follow-up.

Snake Phobia. Hafner (1978) described the treatment of a 25-year-old female with a severe snake phobia by two sessions of prolonged exposure. After reassurance that the speed and duration of exposure would be under her control, the subject underwent *in vivo* exposure to a 1.2-m-long live python. During the four hours of exposure, emotions of anger, grief, guilt, and disgust were as prominent as anxiety and fear. These emotions seemed related to the emergence of vivid mental images that the subject believed were buried memories. During the second session, a cathartic outpouring of grief and rage occurred. This was followed by a period of calm and relaxation, during which exposure proceeded much more rapidly. Hafner states that "these findings suggest that the cathartic or abreactive expression of a range of emotions during exposure therapies such as this may improve outcome, perhaps by facilitating anxiety reduction" (p. 305). Such responses are not unusual. Often symptom-contingent cues result in cathartic reactions "higher on the avoidance hierarchy."

Urinary Retention. Two clients with chronic psychogenic urinary retention were treated by flooding *in vivo* (Antman, 1973). They were exposed to the inhibiting stimulus of urinating in a lavatory outside the home without avoidance or escape permitted; they could not leave the toilet until they passed urine. Initially it took Subject A 2 hr and Subject B ½ hr to urinate. Both improved rapidly; one was treated in 8 sessions, and one required 13 sessions. Despite some residual difficulties, both subjects had maintained their gains at the 9-month follow-up.

Obsessive-Compulsive. An *in vivo* flooding technique was employed with a 25-year-old male with chronic obsessive-compulsive behavior (McCarthy, 1972). The client engaged in ritualistic decontamination that had progressed to the point where he spent 16 hr a day washing himself and his belongings. The year 1957 was significant in the compulsive behavior, so the therapist instructed the client to secure a coin and a map from the year 1957 and to touch these items frequently. Ritualistic behavior and obsessive thoughts extinguished within 48 hr and an 18-month follow-up indicated that the client had remained symptom-free. McCarthy also described the successful use of implosive therapy in treating obsessive fears. Incapacitating symptoms of a 20-year-old male undergraduate were ameliorated following four sessions of implosive therapy.

Escalator Phobia. An escalator phobia of seven years duration was successfully treated in one session of flooding *in vivo* (Nesbitt, 1973). The client was required to ride up and down on escalators with the therapist. After 27 min, she was able to ride alone and after 29 min, the session was terminated because the client felt she no longer needed treatment. A 6-month follow-up indicated that the approach behavior had been maintained and that the client no longer experienced debilitating anxiety approaching or riding an escalator.

Firearm Phobia. A 43-year-old policeman developed a firearm phobia following an incident in which he was shot at. The phobia had not improved during one year of conventional psychotherapy and pharmacotherapy. The avoidance behavior was subsequently treated with *in vivo* flooding combined with motor activity, modeling, and social reinforcement (Naud, Boisvert, & Lamontagne, 1973). After 66 min of flooding, behavioral and physiological measurements showed a trend toward symptom reduction (extinction). The same measurements taken one week after treatment indicated the same trend. At a 5-month follow-up, the patient was still free from his specific phobia; free-floating anxiety remained a problem.

Sharp Object Phobia. Sammah (1975) used flooding to extinguish chronic fear-producing thoughts, homicidal-suicidal thoughts, and depressive behavior in a 45-year-old psychotic female. Although the patient had not responded to 10 years of traditional psychotherapy and drug treatment, she was successfully treated by 10 sessions of behavior therapy. Behavioral techniques included flooding to overcome obsessional fears of knives and other sharp objects, thought-stopping, and reciprocal reinforcements. At the beginning of therapy, the patient was unable to approach sharp objects and reacted with extreme anxiety and screaming at the sight of a knife; with flooding, her fear was reduced to the point where she was able to use knives and other sharp tools in an appropriate manner. Therapy was followed by maintenance telephone calls. The patient had not relapsed at the 20-month follow-up.

Posttraumatic Stress Disorder. Keane and Kaloupek (1982) treated a 36-year-old Vietnam veteran for a posttraumatic stress disorder secondary to a traumatic war experience of 14 years earlier. The veteran suffered from chronic anxiety and depression, frequent nightmares that relived traumatic war events, flashbacks to war events, alcohol abuse, social alienation, and vocational problems. He was treated with 19 sessions of imaginal flooding over a 22-day hospitalization period. Reduction of anxiety and anxiety symptoms (e.g., nightmares, flashbacks) was documented by extensive measurements of heart rate and by systematic self-report data. These changes, as well as improved overall adjustment (e.g., drinking, work), were maintained over a 10-month follow-up period. Similarly, Fairbank and Keane (1981) used imaginal flooding to decrease anxiety (as measured by self-report, heart rate, and skin conductance response) in two Vietnam veterans suffering a posttraumatic stress disorder. Furthermore, the extinction of anxiety to one traumatic memory generalized to other memories only to the extent that the memories shared common elements. This result is consistent with learning theory and suggests, especially when events are dissimilar, the importance of identifying and independently treating each traumatic event.

Techniques Using Variations of Flooding or Implosive Therapy

Self-Implosion. Zimmerman (1975) reported on three subjects who used "self-implosion" or homework alone to modify negative feelings. Each subject used a wrist counter to record the frequency of aversive feelings during baseline, treatment, and follow-up. Subject 1 worked on "hurt feelings": whenever she experienced hurt, she counted it and, as soon as she was alone, "self-imploded." She fantasized rejection, humiliation, and other hurtful situations until the hurt diminished. Subject 2 had feelings of jealously that were interfering with his relationship with his girlfriend. In situations that caused him to feel jealous, his self-implosion consisted of his imagining the worst possible consequences occurring. Subject 3 had a severe driving phobia; she was able to apply self-implosion while driving and experiencing anxiety. All three subjects improved.

Implosion with Hypnosis. The use of implosive therapy with hypnosis may be indicated when resistance to imagery exposure is so extreme that the client is unable to generate anxiety when presented with an image. In such cases, the concomitant use of hypnosis and implosive therapy has been reported to result in swift and often dramatic improvement. Boudewyns and Wilson (1972) routinely used hypnosis with implosive therapy to achieve successful results.

O'Donnell (1978) described a 29-year-old female with a severe and incapacitating cancer phobia who was treated during one week with 3-hour-long sessions of implosive therapy under hypnosis. Behavioral and subjective rating scales completed prior to, during, and following treatment for up to 8 months revealed a significant decrease in phobic anxiety and hypochondriacal behavior. Wijesinghe (1974) reported a case study of a 24-year-old female with a vomiting phobia of 11 years duration that had worsened during the previous 18 months. In the first two sessions, images failed to produce an anxiety response; during the third session, the client was instructed in hypnosis. Following one session of flooding under a hypnotic trance, the phobia was ameliorated. The client was seen on a supportive basis every two weeks for three months and improvement continued. Follow-up a year later indicated that she remained free of her phobia.

Use of Tape Recordings. Implosive clients are routinely assigned homework between therapy sessions. Generally, they are instructed to expose themselves repeatedly to phobic stimuli, either *in vivo* or in fantasy. Tape recordings are frequently used to facilitate imagery exposure homework. Denholtz (1970) feels that tapes can also be used *during* therapy sessions to reduce the strain on the therapist. He presented a case study of a male with premature ejaculation and fears of paternity and homosexuality who was treated with a tape-recorded flooding procedure. After the second session, the client was given the tape to play at home twice a day. Within two weeks, his sexual anxiety had decreased, and he was able to have sex successfully with a new partner.

A 45-year-old hospitalized female with depression, anorexia, and conversion symptoms was treated with tape-recorded implosive therapy (Beutler, 1973). Since the patient was unaware of stimuli that produced symptoms, the therapist used Freudian theory to generate scenes. Scenes were recorded and given to the patient to play on the ward. The treatment lasted 15 days and was successful in ameliorating the symptoms. A 6-month follow-up revealed only one recurrence of hysterical symptoms, and at 12 months the patient reported no further symptoms and indicated that she was married and was working full-time.

Stambaugh (1977) reported the successful treatment of incapacitating somatic problems in a 28-year-old male with the use of two tape-recorded flooding scenarios. Not only were the somatic problems alleviated, but the client also began behaving more assertively and was able to discontinue the use of antianxiety medications. At 1-month and 1-year follow-ups, there was indication that therapeutic gains were maintained.

Pinto (1972) reported the successful flooding treatment of a 31-year-old male with agoraphobia. The man had had movement-induced seizures since the age of seven, with seizure frequency increasing during times of stress. He began to fear that he would have seizures in public and subsequently developed agoraphobia. During treatment, he listened to tape-recorded fantasies in which he was pictured as entering intensely phobic situations and developing seizures, with all the feared embarrassment. The scenes were repeated until the fantasy ceased to evoke anxiety. Immediately afterward, the patient went into the situation just fantasied, such as crossing a street or entering a store. Treatment consisted of 10 fantasy sessions each followed by 10 *in vivo* practice sessions. At discharge, the patient had no difficulty traveling. Although the flooding was instituted primarily to treat the agoraphobia, it was hoped that some improvement would occur in the frequency of seizures that seemed related to the degree of anxiety the patient was experiencing at the time. After treatment began, the patient had no seizures, and at the end of the last two sessions, he was unable to produce a seizure when urged to do so. He remained seizure-free at the 16-week follow-up.

Flooding and Implosive Therapy with Children

Flooding and implosive therapy have been effective in the treatment of anxiety-related problems in children. Evidence is primarily anecdotal and no controlled studies have been conducted in this age group. However, case studies report that beneficial effects occur rapidly and follow-up data indicate that therapeutic gains are maintained.

Yule, Sacks, and Hersov (1974) reported the treatment of an 11-year-old boy with a severe phobia for loud noises. Although *in vivo* desensitization had been unsuccessful, two sessions of *in vivo* flooding, in which the boy burst balloons, successfully alleviated the phobia. Over a

25-month follow-up period, the boy continued to be free of the phobic behavior.

Smith and Sharpe (1970) employed implosive therapy in the treatment of a 13-year-old boy who had been suffering from a school phobia of two months duration. Following one session, the boy was able to return to school and attend his most anxiety-arousing class. After four sessions, he was able to return to school on a full-time basis with only fleeting anxiety. Follow-up data revealed that the boy not only had remained free of anxiety but had also shown substantial improvement in school grades and peer relationships.

Ollendick and Gruen (1972) presented the case study of an 8-year-old boy with a 3-year history of a pervasive fear of bleeding to death following injury. The bodily injury phobia developed following the birth of a retarded sister who had a disorder in which her blood would not clot. The boy had also been removed from his parent's room at this time. The phobia was expressed in the behavioral symptoms of sleepless nights (averaging 5 to 7 nights per week), asthmatic bronchitis, and hives (allergy testing was negative). Following two sessions of imaginal implosive therapy, the number of sleepless nights for the boy diminished to two per week, and there was no recurrence of hives or asthmatic bronchitis during treatment or at a 6-month follow-up. Further follow-up revealed a complete remission of sleepless nights and improvement in peer relationships and self-concept.

Finally, the youngest child reported in the literature to be treated with flooding was a 4-year-old boy with extreme social withdrawal (Kandel, Ayllon, & Rosenbaum, 1977). A within-subject design, consisting of multiple baselines across settings, was employed. Several children provided social stimuli. When flooding was introduced in the first setting, a dramatic increase in interaction from 0 to 60% occurred, with an accompanying decrease in self-talk from 70 to 20%. These behavioral changes did not occur in the second setting until flooding was introduced. With the flooding technique, interaction increased from 10 to 40% and self-talk decreased from 85 to 20%. The 5-month follow-up indicated that therapeutic gains were maintained.

4

THEORY AND TECHNIQUE

Implosive Therapy: Theory and Technique

Thomas Stampfl originally developed implosive therapy based, in part, on Mowrer's two-factor theory (Mowrer, 1960). Two-factor theory suggests that stimuli paired with pain or deprivation come to elicit negative emotions. These emotions, in turn, motivate defensive maneuvers. Maneuvers that successfully reduce or terminate the feared conditioned stimuli are reinforced by the reduction in negative affect. Continued symptomatic avoidance of stimuli that elicit negative affect prevents extinction from occurring. In implosive therapy, the client is repeatedly exposed to those stimuli he or she has learned to fear. It is the repetition of these avoided stimuli in the absence of physical pain or deprivation that leads to a progressive reduction in the emotional responses that drive the symptomatic behavior of the patient. Reduction or elimination of this drive state leads to a reduction or elimination of the patient's avoidance symptoms.

Extinction of negative emotions is assumed to be a function of the number and duration of exposures to previously conditioned aversive stimuli (Shipley, 1974). Therefore, when a client reacts to a portion of the imagined scene, it is essential that those cues be repeated again and again. Since the therapist cannot ascertain which of the presented cues approximate the originally conditioned cues, the theme that produces the emotional reaction is expanded to cover a range of stimuli, thus allowing generalization of extinction. For example, a client who fears expressing anger to his employer is repeatedly instructed to imagine doing so with his most dire fears of retaliation and rejection confirmed. He is also directed to imagine expressing extreme anger toward his co-workers, wife, parents, therapist, and others, as long as such imagery evokes relatively strong emotion. Each aspect of a scene is repeated until it no longer elicits emotion.

Task of the Therapist

The fundamental task of the implosive therapist is to reproduce repeatedly (usually through imagery) those stimulus situations to which anxiety responses have been conditioned. By exposing the client to the stimulus situations that are being avoided or escaped, the full emotional impact associated with those cues will be experienced. It has been debated whether anxiety is necessary for extinction or just an unfortunate by-product of CS exposure. Regardless, in implosive therapy, one of the therapist's prime goals is to present repeatedly material which elicits anxiety or other negative emotions so that negative affect is *ultimately* extinguished. In the absence of any primary reinforcement, a marked reduction in the negative emotional state should occur with continued repetition of the CS complex. Once the motivating source for maintaining the client's symptoms is sufficiently reduced, the symptoms will cease to be elicited. Thus, the therapist is not attempting merely to induce anxiety but also to reproduce those stimulus patterns with their secondary drive properties that are thought to provide the motivational force for the symptomatology. To this end, the implosive therapist has two primary duties. First, he must conduct "detective work" to delineate those cues, (both obvious and hypothesized) that produce emotional upset in the client and result in avoidance behavior, and second he must direct implosive scenes for the client to imagine or experience.

The Therapist–Client Relationship

The only exposure many therapists have had to implosive therapy has been the viewing or hearing of a portion of a therapy session during which a client is bombarded with vivid descriptions of terrifying, disgusting, or otherwise aversive scenes. With this limited exposure, it is no wonder that many therapists have negative opinions of this technique. It is true that during the implosive scenes the therapist is directive and unsympathetic in demanding that the client visualize scenes that cause emotional discomfort. However, the presentation of scenes represents only one of two distinctly different levels of communication between therapist and client. When a scene is not being presented, the therapist is very supportive, recognizing the suffering of the client and reinforcing the client's courage in imagining the scenes.

Furthermore, the more sensitive and empathetic the therapist is in understanding the client's problem, the better he or she will be able to present relevant material. The maintenance of a supportive therapist–client relationship is as essential, if not more essential, in implosive therapy as in any other form of treatment. Therefore, it is important for the therapist to emphasize that, when the client closes his eyes and imagines a scene, he is in one aspect of therapy and when he opens his eyes and interacts with the therapist, he is in another. This dual process of communication removes the therapist from the aversive scenes, reducing negative feelings toward the therapist for exposing the client to anxiety-producing material, and helps the client to discriminate the various roles of the therapist.

The dual process of communication has another function. The imagined attitudes and behaviors of the client are to be accepted as true while the fantasy is in progress. However, no inference is made by the therapist that implications from the imagined scenes constitute an accurate reflection of the client's attitudes or behaviors. Thus, the client is asked to believe the implications for a given behavior in one mode of communication with the therapist (during scene presentation) but need not accept them in the other mode. If a client reports that some of the imagined material is actually true, the therapist has the option to agree, disagree, or remain neutral.

Informed Consent

The client should be provided with an explanation of the theoretical basis of implosive therapy and the procedure that will be followed. Not only does such an explanation meet the ethical and legal requirement of informed consent, but it also facilitates the client's cooperation. The language used in the explanation should be clear and understandable by the particular client. An example of how such information may be provided is stated here:

> You have learned to be anxious in certain situations through past traumatic experiences in similar situations, or through seeing or hearing about the traumatic experiences of others. Regardless of how you learned to be fearful, your other symptoms (such as ritualistic behavior, phobic avoidance, nonassertion) are ways of avoiding exposing yourself to those things you fear. Your avoidance behaviors prevent you from feeling anxious. However, if we could remove your fears, the other symptoms (avoidance behaviors) would drop out. Let me give you an example. If your child almost drowned, he might learn to fear the water and consequently would avoid water. He might also fear the beach and anything else associated with his traumatic experience. If your child is successful

in avoiding all contact with water, it is likely that he will maintain his fear over the years. What would you do to help your child overcome his fear of the water? (The client generally gives an answer which recognizes that some repetitious exposure to the feared situation would be required.) Yes, repeated exposure to water until the learned fear is "unlearned" would be needed. This type of treatment is similar to the old saying that if a horse throws you, you should get right back on the horse to prevent the development of a fear and an avoidance of horses.

How would you expose your child to the water? Gradually or all at once? To expose him gradually, you could first convince him to sit on the beach and then instruct him to move nearer and nearer to the water; then to put his big toe in the water; then his foot and so on, making certain that his fear was abated at each point in the exposure before proceeding to the next step, until the child gradually overcame his fear of the water. An alternative approach would be to persuade or force your child to jump in the water and remain there until his fear subsided. The gradual exposure has the advantage of subjecting the child to less intense fear, but it would probably require a much greater amount of time for fear reduction to occur than the all-at-once approach. The more complicated and pervasive a person's fears, the more crucial is the treatment time factor.

We have treatments for avoidance behaviors that are similar to those you might use with a child afraid of water. Since most people's fears are less concrete and more complicated than the fear of water, rather than participate in the "real life" situation, we have the person close his eyes and imagine a feared scene directed by the therapist. We can do this either gradually or all at once. I would personally recommend the all-at-once strategy because this approach generally produces faster results. However, it would require a lot of work on your part and perhaps a good deal of emotional discomfort. It would involve your imagining anxiety-producing scenes here in the office and a couple of times each day at home. What do you think? (The client usually has questions to direct to the therapist.)

If the client agrees to participate in this type of therapy, the diagnostic detective work is begun. Prior to this, however, therapists may find it useful to obtain baseline measures of adjustment/symptoms for diagnostic purposes and to help evaluate therapeutic outcome.

Detective Work

The therapist attempts to discover the internal and external stimuli that elicit negative emotions (such as anxiety, depression, guilt or anger) or defensive maneuvers designed to avoid negative emotions. In order to do this, the therapist must continually ask, "What are the conditioned cues that the client is avoiding?" From theory, it is assumed that these cues are multiple, involve a variety of stimuli, may be historical in origin, and are ordered sequentially or serially in terms of avoidance strength and accessibility. Those environmental or situational cues that are determined to be highly correlated with the occurrence of the client's symptoms (symptom-contingent cues) and that are readily identifiable by the client are considered to have less of an anxiety loading. The symptom-contingent cues, however, are not expected to reflect all the cues responsible for motivating symptom formation. Hence, elimination of these cues is usually only a first step. Other cues, stored in the memory and recoverable as the anxiety associated with symptom-contingent cues is reduced, are ordered in a sequential fashion in terms of aversive loading—the more aversive cues are assumed to be closer in time to the historical events during which the original unconditioned stimulus was presented. On exposure, these cues are assumed to be capable of eliciting considerably higher levels of anxiety than symptom-contingent cues. If responses to these early cues are not extinguished, they have the potential to become reassociated with other stimuli and to initiate other avoidance patterns. By using the theoretical construct, the Avoidance Serial Cue Hierarchy (Stampfl & Levis, 1967), the therapist attempts to identify the cues responsible for motivating the avoidance behavior. Stampfl and Levis (1966) have delineated four types of cues.

Symptom-Contingent Cues. These cues are directly related to the occurrence of increased negative affect or increased instrumental avoidance tendencies by the client. They can generally be deduced by analyzing the contingencies surrounding the occurrence of the symptom. They are accessible and identifiable by the client and are assumed to have less of an anxiety loading than cues higher on the Avoidance Serial Cue Hierarchy. Neurotic phobic reactions represent the most obvious example of this type of cue. Avoidance tendencies are augmented by the proximity to the phobic object or situation and unavoidable exposure increases negative affect. Thus, external features of the phobic object or situation become symptom-contingent cues. Compulsive reactions also exemplify responses to symptom-contingent cues.

Reportable Internally Elicited Cues. Related to symptom-contingent cues are internal responses reportable by the client that appear to have aversive properties. For example, for an acrophobic, a high place represents a symptom-contingent cue. However, the covert stimuli associated with the client's thoughts of falling, bodily mutilation, and death comprise internally elicited cues. Such cues have been reported by clients with a diverse range of maladaptive behavioral reactions and, on questioning, clients are frequently able to supply detailed descriptions of cues classifiable under this category. For example, the claustrophobic may report a fear of suffocation and relate the fear with marginal thoughts that he is being punished; the compulsive handwasher may associate his behavior with thoughts of being dirty and with vague feelings of guilt. These types of cues appear to be present in most every client, both neurotic and psychotic.

Unreportable Cues Hypothesized to Relate to Reportable Internally Elicited Cues. These cues are hypothesized by the therapist to have a logical relationship to symptom-contingent and reportable cues. The therapist may determine them by analyzing the conditioning history of the client and making assumptions about the critical features of the conditioning process. For example, much aversive conditioning is assumed to be associated with the fear of bodily injury (dying from infection, falling from a tall building, being hit by a car, being cut). Even if not reported by the client, the therapist can assume that stimuli directly associated with tissue injury are integral elements of the aversive stimulus complex. Thus, the client who fears falling from a high place also fears the bodily consequences of the impact following the fall. Stimuli associated with the client's mangled body are a logical consequence of the aversive sequence related to the phobia: S_1, high places; S_2, falling; S_3, impact; S_4, blood and other stimuli associated with a mangled body; S_5, death.

Based on experience, other common hypothesized cues center around the expression of hostility and aggression toward parental figures, punishment or retaliation for transgressive behavior by the client, and cues related to experiences of sex, shame, guilt, rejection, deprivation, abandonment, and helplessness. Hypothesized cues may include the stimulus characteristics of events inferred by the therapist to have existed in the conditioning history or actually reported by the client to have occurred.

Hypothesized Dynamic Cues. Hypothesized dynamic cues are derived from psychoanalytically based theories of personality, tend to be more completely avoided or repressed by the client, and can be deduced from hypothetical events in early conditioning experiences. The use of dynamic cues is probably one of the more controversial aspects of implosive therapy, but many therapists have found Freudian source material helpful in generating hypothesized cues (see, for example, Fenichel, 1945), and these cues appear to be especially useful in the treatment of more severely disturbed clients. Freudian theory would suggest, for example, the consideration of "toileting" scenes with severely obsessive-compulsive individuals or "infantile sexuality" and "masturbation" scenes with persons presenting with conversion hysteria.

More recently, Levis and Hare (1977) revised the cue categories with the aim of increasing operational specificity. They described seven categories and suggested that this classification system is more beneficial for indicating the kinds of material that ought to be introduced into therapy. Whereas flooding treatments generally involve only the first two categories, implosive techniques may involve any of the seven cue categories.

Inherently Nonharmful Situational and Environmental Cues (CSs) Preceding Symptom Onset and Believed Correlated with It. These cues include those that initiate symptoms but precede the actual avoidance behavior. For a person who fears heights, viewing a tall building from the ground would be classified in this category.

Inherently Nonharmful Situational Environmental Cues (CSs) Directly Avoided by Symptom Onset. These cues are those that are partially or completely avoided by symptom onset and that have a high probability of occurring if avoidance behavior is not activated. Examples include riding elevators, looking out of windows, and being assertive. Categories one and two are comparable to the symptom-contingent cues.

Physically Harmful Cues (USs) Hypothesized to Be Anticipated Given the Failure of Symptom Onset. These cues are hypothesized by the therapist as representing aversive unconditioned consequences of the feared situation that are ameliorated by symptom onset. For instance, to the individual afraid of tall buildings, the fear of bodily injury following a fall from a high place would be classified in this category. For the individual who fears flying, it is likely that his greatest fear is not the situational cues associated with flying in an airplane *per se* but that the plane will crash and he will be injured or killed. Implosive therapists consider these cues to be vital to treatment and they can be logically deduced from analyzing the symptoms. Consequently, in developing imaginal scenes, the therapist generally depicts the worst possible event that could happen when the client participates in the feared situation.

Hypothesized External Environmental Cues Deduced to Be Associated with the Original (Historical) Conditioning Sequences. These cues include those events that are likely to have occurred during the past (generally during early childhood) and contributed to the development of symptom formation. Experiences dealing with sex, punishment, rejection, guilt, bodily injury, illness, and religion may be presented. These cues may be hypothesized by the therapist (based on interview material or on assumptions about the conditioning history of the client) or recalled during treatment.

Hypothesized Internal Thought Processes Deduced to Be Associated with the Original (Historical) Conditioning Sequences. These cues include the internal thought processes associated with the external conditioning events; they also become conditioned, are historical in origin, and generally involve the elicitation of strong emotions that are usually considered taboo. If a male client was severely beaten by his father for masturbating as a small child, internalized cues associated with the original conditioning may also include fear of castration and perhaps the desire to kill the father.

Hypothesized Stimulus Generalization Equivalent to the Presenting Phobic Stimulus. This category includes cues that may be related symbolically to the phobic stimulus. For example, the phobic stimulus of a knife may be symbolic and may be related to a phobia involving the penis. This category is primarily useful in research to test hypotheses concerning symptom formation.

Hypothesized Avoided Cues Eliciting Emotional Reactions Other Than Those Represented by the Label of Fear or Anxiety. These cues involve emotions other than fear and anxiety and may include feelings of love, happiness, and anger. Scenes would be presented depicting assertiveness, successfulness and love in an effort to extinguish avoidance behaviors that inhibit these emotions.

Therapeutic Programming and Initial Diagnostic Interviews

The "detective work" that continues throughout therapy is initiated by conducting two or three diagnostic interviews. The initial interviews cover the material generally gathered in taking a clinical psychosocial case history (Lieb, Lipsitch, & Slaby, 1973). Particular attention, however, is focused on the stimulus determinants of current symptomatic behavior, past traumatic events, childhood fears, and repetitive aversive dreams.

Stimuli that immediately precede the client's negative emotions and symptomatic behavior are explored in detail, with the therapist searching for common stimulus elements. Take, for example, a client who is experiencing acute anxiety attacks. If the client experienced one attack while driving, the therapist would make a detailed inquiry into the external and internal stimuli present prior to the attack—who was with the client, the time of day, the weather conditions, where the client was going, road stimuli such as bridges or hills, what the radio was playing, and, most importantly, what the client was thinking. In order to determine potential internal-avoided stimuli, the client is asked to imagine and report the worse possible thing that could happen in the feared situation. If the anxiety attack occurred while driving alone at night on wet pavement, the client might report the fear of losing control of the car. The therapist then asks what could be the worst thing that might happen if the client lost control of the car. If the client reports that he or she might be in an accident and die, the therapist would follow up by inquiring about the worst aspects of such a death—pain and bodily injury, being alone, punishment in hell for past misdeeds. The therapist would also determine whether the client experiences a fear of loss of control in other situations. Each occurrence of symptomatic behavior would be explored in a similar fashion. The therapist must continually ask himself, "What does the client fear? What are the external and internal conditioned cues that the client is avoiding?" and then look for commonalities across these situations.

Past Traumatic Events. Neutral stimuli, when paired in time with pain or deprivation, become capable of eliciting negative emotions. Therefore, the therapist inquires about early aversive events in the client's history that may have been conditioning experiences. Prominent among these experiences are parental punishment practices. The therapist asks what types of behaviors (aggression, sexual behavior, toileting behavior, nonachievement) lead to punishment; what types of punishment (verbal reprimand, spanking, isolation) were administered and by whom; and what the client's reactions to the punishments were. Illness, accidents, fights, and other presumed traumatic events are also explored for stimulus similarities to the situations currently eliciting symptomatic behavior.

Childhood Fears. Although most young children experience some fears, inquiry into the childhood fears of the client occasionally reveals unusual or protracted fears that appear to be directly related to current symptoms.

Repetitive Aversive Dreams. Repetitive nightmares generally include stimulus elements similar to the stimulus determinants of the client's symptomatic behavior. For example, a man who had been in a tornado, had recurring dreams of being trapped in a violent storm. Since this man was a construction worker and often worked outside, he had been unable to work for five years due to his fear of bad weather. The client also experienced repetitive nightmares of being chased by the police. This dream suggested that he felt guilty and feared punishment for his sins and/or that he felt that people were out to get him. Further inquiry into his history revealed that, even prior to his traumatic experience with tornadoes, he had never held a job for more than six months because he developed paranoid feelings about his co-workers. Furthermore, he revealed incidences of misbehavior that led both to his guilt feelings and to the projection of anger onto others. Because of the information collected through the detective work, implosive scenes utilized in this case not only recreated the tornadoes and their feared consequences of injury and death, but also exposed the client to his previous misbehavior and the resulting guilt and feared punishment.

Past Successful Scenes. One source of implosive scene material that is not generated by direct questioning or observation of the client is the use of past successful scenes. As an implosive therapist gains experience treating clients with particular problems, he frequently discovers a common scene or scenes that elicit emotions in these clients. The therapist may subsequently introduce some variant of these scenes to clients presenting with similar symptoms. For example, clients exhibiting fear of interpersonal rejection and separation might be directed to imagine the "baby-in-the-crib" scene. In this scene the client visualizes himself as an infant in a crib. He is alone, tired, wet, cold, hungry, thirsty, helpless, and in need of touch. All of his needs are unmet and he is crying for his mother. After a long time, his mother finally enters the room and takes out her breast as if to give him nourishment, warmth, touch, and caring. The client's hopes are raised and he thinks his mother will take care of his needs. Then the mother is pictured as squirting her milk on the floor, screaming her hatred for the client, and leaving him alone in the crib to suffer and die. The test of the scene's relevance to a particular client lies in the individual reaction—those parts of the scene that elicit a strong emotional reaction are relevant and are expanded and repeated. Other common themes that are relevant to particular problems, such as aggression, rejection, depression, and feelings of inferiority, have been summarized elsewhere (Hogan, 1968; Stampfl & Levis, 1969).

Beginning with the initial interviews, the "detective work" continues throughout the treatment process. Cue usage is constantly modified, based on the client's behavior during and after the presentation of the scenes; if cues elicit anxiety or defensive behavior, the assumption is made that the client has been conditioned to them previously. Furthermore, during each session, the stimulus determinants of symptoms that occurred during the preceding week are explored as are any repetitive dreams. Thus, the treatment plan and the implosive scenes are modified by feedback from the client.

Emotion during a Scene. The client's level of emotion during a particular portion of an implosive scene is assumed to indicate the salience of the stimuli being presented. One client became highly anxious when the therapist instructed him to imagine himself as a youth taking a shower at the local YMCA with other boys. This stimulus complex was assumed to contain at least some relevant conditioned stimuli. On the basis of this feedback, the therapist expanded and repeated aspects of the shower room scene and, following the scene, asked the client about shower-room and related experiences.

Imagery during a Scene. Anxiety is considered to be the mediator of image clarity (Haney & Euse, 1976). Therefore, the client's ability to form a mental image during various portions of a scene can be used diagnostically. If a portion of an implosive scene is pictured clearly without anxiety, it is assumed to be irrelevant to the client's problem; if it is pictured clearly with anxiety, it is thought to be relevant. However, if a client with generally good imagery reports being unable to imagine particular stimulus events, this difficulty is viewed as an avoidance response and the avoided material is assumed to be highly relevant. Occasionally, to overcome resistance, a more graded exposure to highly charged scenes may be necessary. For example, a woman whose husband frequently worked nights presented with extreme fear of staying alone at night. When asked what the worst thing that could happen in this situation would be, she answered that someone might break into the house and beat her up. Other interview material suggested that the client might desire other sexual contacts and that she feared this desire. An implosive scene was introduced that pictured her home alone at night; she hears a noise; a man breaks into her house, beats her, drags her to the bedroom, rapes her, and she responds lustily. During the initial presentation of this scene, the client was able to visualize, with accompanying anxiety, all but the sexual portions of the scene. Her inability to imagine the sexual scene was supportive of the hypothesis that sexual stimuli were important elicitors of anxiety in need of exposure. With repetition, the anxiety generated by this portion of the scene diminished and the client was gradually able to visualize and experience the fear associated, first, with the rape scene, and, finally, with her sexual response to the imagined sexual attack. Thus, if a client is unable to picture particular aspects of a scene, these aspects are considered to be very strong elicitors of anxiety—strong enough to motivate the avoidance maneuver of reduced image clarity.

Recovery of Forgotten Material. Sometimes following a scene, the client reports remembering a past traumatic event. Such memories generally relate to the content of the just-completed scene and provide relevant material for future scenes. For example, a man being treated for impotence was asked to imagine an early traumatic incidence of erection failure. Following the scene, the client reported remembering an incident that occurred when he was in the first grade. The teacher asked him to write the numbers one through ten on the blackboard and, although he felt he knew how to do so, he was unable to write the number six. His inability to write this number resulted in his experiencing extreme ridicule from the female teacher before his classmates. This memory provided material for subsequent implosive scenes.

Neutral Scene Presentation

Following the initial "detective work" to generate hypotheses regarding the cues that the client is avoiding and prior to the presentation of implosive scenes, one or more neutral scenes are presented to the client.

The client is instructed to close his eyes and to imagine the scenes that the therapist directs. It is best to begin with a familiar and stationary scene, for instance, the exterior of the client's home. Then the client is instructed to begin moving into the environment, always emphasizing that the client is an active participant and not merely a viewer in the fantasy. The therapist directs the fantasy and asks the client to provide descriptions. The therapist might simply say, "Now you're entering the living room; feel yourself walking through the door, pushing the door open; feel the pressure on your hand. Look in the room and see the furniture. Look around the room and describe the room to me." From the client's description, the therapist gets feedback on the strength of visual imagery. Does the client provide a detailed or a cursory description? The therapist should encourage the client to go into detail. It is important for the client to respond in imagery with all senses—sight, smell, taste, touch, hearing—allowing the therapist to question the client about sounds, smells, or textures in the living room and later in other scenes. If the client is able to visualize clearly the living room scene, he is next asked to imagine a scene that includes events which could never happen. For example, the client may be asked to imagine himself standing by a stream on a pleasant spring day, to notice the landscape, the trees beside him, the colors and smells, to feel the warmth of the sun, and to hear the gurgling of the stream. He is then instructed to imagine looking up in the sky and seeing a bird glide and soar, and wishing that he could be a bird. He then looks down and watches his arms change into wings and he is able to fly like a bird. The therapist directs the client to imagine all aspects of flying—the breeze blowing over his body, the feeling of freedom, the feeling of gliding and soaring. The client views the world from the sky for a time and then returns to land by the stream. His wings are changed back into arms and he is asked to open his eyes. An inquiry is then conducted into the intensity and quality of the imagery.

The use of neutral imagery accomplishes four things:

1. *It provides the therapist with a crude baseline of the client's ability to use imagery.* Some clients have little visual imagery, but this is very rare, occurring in 5% or less of clients. If problems are experienced during these initial neutral scenes, the client is asked to practice the scenes at least twice a day for the next week. Frequently, clients show improvement in their ability to image as a result of such practice.
2. *The therapist is established as director of the scenes.* It is important that the client allow the therapist to control the content of the scenes, since later he will be asked to imagine unpleasant scenes that may produce resistance.
3. *The neutral scene demonstrates the possibility of imagining things that have never happened or could never happen.* The therapist emphasizes

that when the client closes his eyes, he is imagining events that may or may not be possible. This is important since a client will occasionally say that he cannot imagine something presented in an implosive scene (for example, beating his wife) because he has never experienced that event before. The therapist can then gently challenge the client by noting that he has never flown like a bird but was able to imagine doing so in the neutral scene.

4. *The neutral scene can be used to help teach the client that events occurring in fantasy are not "real."* The client can experience *anything* in fantasy, and visual imagery can be very useful in reducing fears about cues in which *in vivo* scenes would not be practical. Thus, in fantasy, a client can fall from a tall building, suffer bodily injury, die and be condemned to hell, but when he opens his eyes and comes back to reality, he realizes that "nothing has happened."

Implosive Sessions

After establishing a warm therapist–client relationship, discovering the cues thought to generate emotional responses and symptoms, and practicing imagery with neutral scenes, the actual treatment sessions may begin. The client is encouraged to be a good "actor" during the implosive scenes, to try to "live" the scene and to experience the relevant emotions as if the scene were actually happening. He is to picture the scenes not as an onlooker but rather as if he were directly and personally involved. He is reminded that he need not accept the imagined attitudes and behaviors as existing within the "real" world, but should try to accept them fully within the fantasy, just as an actor would accept a role.

Timing of Cue Presentation. As discussed earlier, several types of cues are thought to be ordered on an Avoidance Serial Cue Hierarchy, from least to most avoided. The implosive therapist must make a tactical decision regarding which type of stimuli to present first and which to present last. Concrete symptom-contingent cues that elicit anxiety (such as seeing a tall building, a crowd, or a snake) and the associated reportable internal cues (such as fear of suffocation reported by the claustrophobic) are usually presented first. These cues are easily accessible to the client and readily respond to implosive treatment. Hypothesized fears that are further from the client's awareness have a greater aversive loading; such fears are more difficult to extinguish and are dealt with last. For example, a client may fear an external stimulus such as crowds, not because of an aversive experience with crowds, but because the stimuli of crowds are associated with feared internal stimuli.

These internal cues may include fears that the people in the crowd will attack and injure the client or that the client will attack people in the crowd. It is also possible that the client fears confessing his or her sins to them or acting-out sexually before them. The symptom-contingent cue of "crowd" is the least feared and would be presented first. The internal hypothesized cues are generally beyond the client's awareness (at least during the initial stages of therapy), and as the most feared cues are presented last.

Establishing the Setting of the Scene. Prior to beginning the implosive scene, the therapist generally prepares an outline of a story-like scene. Frequently, the scene begins as a replay of some past traumatic incident or recurrent dream. The therapist involves the client in the scene by describing the setting of the story and by presenting relatively non-arousing material first. This is particularly helpful with clients who have difficulty imaging or who otherwise are difficult to involve in a scene. For example, the scene introduced to a client who fears crowds may be a football game—the scene begins with the client preparing to leave home for the game, proceeds with him driving toward the stadium, and finally pictures him in the crowd. This relatively gradual approach to the most feared situation allows the client to become emotionally involved with the scenes and provides for the extinction of anticipatory fear.

Scene Presentation. The therapist should approximate as closely as possible the hypothesized traumatic events and reproduce the cues as realistically as possible. The more detailed and dramatic the description, the easier it is for the client to visualize the scene and experience the emotion. It is frequently helpful for the therapist to find out specific names of people and places and other information in order to make the descriptions more detailed. To further increase the realism of the scene, the therapist may provide sound effects and play the verbal roles of other people in the scenes. The client is encouraged to become involved with as many senses as possible. He is frequently asked to verbalize statements in the present tense to other characters in the scene. He may also be asked to make arm movements appropriate to the action in the scene. For example, a client who fears being aggressive may be helped to imagine beating someone if he makes a fist and punches in the air or if he stomps the floor as he imagines stomping some hated or ambivalently regarded person. Care must be taken here that no pain or harm comes to the client with such movement. Thus, a client who begins pounding his fist onto the wooden arm of a chair should instead be instructed to swing into the air or pound a pillow. Any pain experienced during a scene could lead to conditioning rather than extinction.

At each stage of the process, the therapist attempts to evoke the maximal level of emotion to a given scene. When a high level of emotion is experienced, the client is maintained at this level until a diminution of the emotion-eliciting value of the scene occurs. Then the scene is repeatedly presented until it ceases to elicit much anxiety. Variations of the scene are introduced in order to maximize the process of generalization of extinction.

Handling of Avoidance Responses. Presentation of strongly aversive conditioned stimuli in an implosive scene will sometimes motivate the client to attempt avoidance responses. The most frequent avoidance maneuvers during a scene are reduced image clarity and the blocking of negative emotion. When a client says he cannot or will not imagine a particular portion of a scene or experience the emotion, these scenes are considered to be very relevant and the therapist must attempt to overcome the resistance. To override the resistance directly, the therapist may simply direct the client to continue visualizing the scene and increase the tempo of scene description ("John, you *can* see it, don't block it out, you see it." "Whether it's true or not, just imagine it. You can see it; visualize it now.") Or it may be helpful to attribute reduced client responsibility for the imagined action ("You can do it, see yourself hitting your boss. Something snaps in your mind; it's like *you're not yourself.* You start hitting. . ."). The therapist may also emphasize that the scene is just a fantasy ("John, anything can happen in fantasy; it doesn't necessarily mean that it is 'real.' Now I want you to see your wife's face. . . notice her hateful smile. You feel your hand rising to strike her."). Faced with strong resistance, the therapist can also present stimuli of a slightly lesser intensity for a few minutes and then reattempt the presentation of the stronger stimuli. Resisted material may also be initially presented on a symbolic level, that is, lower on the stimulus–generalization gradient. For example, a boy hypothesized to fear attack by his father might be asked to imagine a monster attacking him.

When a client has trouble with image clarity, extra descriptive detail can be provided. The scene can be developed slowly with liberal description of internal and external stimuli in all sense modalities (e.g., color of clothes, arrangement of furniture, smells, tactile sensations). Inclusion of scenes close to reality may also help, especially in the early stages of therapy. For example, beginning a scene with the client picturing himself or herself sitting in the therapist's office and feeling the actual chair he or she is sitting on. When imagery is reported to be unclear despite the therapist's efforts at descriptive detail, the therapist can simply proceed. Generally, considerable anxiety reduction can be obtained from the auditory input alone and the scene becomes clearer with repetition.

Occasionally, resistance occurs on a scale large enough to interfere severely with treatment, for example, by the client repeatedly arriving late for appointments, cancelling appointments, or failing to accomplish homework assignments. When this occurs, the therapist may, of course, attempt to deal with it in the traditional verbal manner, through discussion or labeling. If strong resistance continues, it is assumed that some negative emotion is motivating the resistance. The therapist attempts to uncover the eliciting stimuli for the aversive emotions and subsequently presents implosive scenes to extinguish them. For example, if a client's resistance to implosive therapy is hypothesized to result from anger at the therapist, the client is asked to delineate the things that are found annoying about the therapist or the therapy. The client's statements are then used to generate implosive scenes designed to reduce the emotion motivating the resistance. Thus, individual clients might report that they are upset at the therapist's yelling at them during the scenes and continually directing them to imagine being aggressive with people they love. Such feelings often make the client feel trapped in the therapy session. The client would then be presented with a scene in which the therapist is pictured as doing all of the objectionable things tenfold. The scene continues with the client feeling upset and trapped and attempting to leave the session. The therapist blocks the client's leaving and hits him or her (all in imagery, of course). The client angrily quarrels with the therapist and then beats and kills him. Anger toward the therapist is generally reduced by the presentation of this scene in the office and several times as homework; after the angry feelings are diminished, the client's resistance largely disappears.

Many clients, particularly those with obsessive-compulsive features, fear losing control and going crazy. For such clients, implosive scenes would include loss of control themes. Such clients may resist implosion, fearing the therapy itself will drive them crazy. This resistance can be dealt with by directly imploding this fear. Typically, a scene would be generated in which the therapy drove the patient crazy according to his or her worst fears. This might include the client "losing his or her mind," acting-out sexually, or becoming aggressive. The scene would typically continue with themes of rejection and/or punishment. With sufficient repetition, such exposure generally lessens this form of resistance.

Finally, when an otherwise cooperative client appears unable to become involved emotionally with implosive scenes, the therapist should check his or her medication usage. If the client is taking antianxiety medication, consideration should be given (in collaboration with the client's physician) to reducing or eliminating the medication, or to timing its ingestion so as to interfere less with arousal during scene practice.

Scene Termination. A given scene is usually terminated after some diminution in anxiety is noted. An implosive scene should not be terminated while a client is emotionally distraught nor should a scene be terminated in the middle of a given scene theme. Following the last scene in a session, the therapist should allow at least 10 minutes to elapse to insure that the client's anxiety level has returned to normal. Experience indicates that no matter how much anxiety is generated during a session, clients generally return to presession or lower anxiety within about a 5-minute period after opening their eyes. Following each scene, an inquiry is made into the vividness of the client's imagery and the amount of emotion experienced during various portions of the scene. The client should report feeling tired and "wrung out" but not anxious. If he feels highly tense, the scene was terminated prematurely. Although premature scene termination should not negate the extinction that has taken place in the scene, it deprives the client of the reinforcement of immediate anxiety reduction. During the first several sessions, it is especially important that the client's anxiety be reduced at scene termination in order to assure his cooperation in future scenes. If for some reason the client's anxiety does not subside quickly, the therapist can focus on a small aspect of the scene and repeat it several times until the emotion attached to that portion of the scene is extinguished. Repetition is the key to anxiety reduction. In subsequent therapy sessions, the more general scene can be repeatedly presented.

Homework Scenes. Following each session, the client is instructed to reenact in imagination at least one homework scene. Typically, the scene assigned is the one just presented during the treatment session and client's may be given a tape of the scene to facilitate their practice. Clients are asked to find a quiet place where they will not be disturbed and to imagine the prescribed scene(s) at least twice daily; usually practice of 20–50 minutes a day is recommended. The client will probably be unable to elicit the same anxiety as the therapist can, but nonetheless is asked to keep track of image clarity and the amount of emotion produced (Wolpe's 0–100 subjective anxiety scale is used for this). These homework scenes are crucial since they provide the repetitive stimulus exposure necessary for the reduction of negative emotions. Therapy time can be greatly reduced if the client is motivated to practice at home. The homework scenes also help to teach the client the technique of implosive therapy so that these techniques can be used as a coping skill for relevant new problems in the client's life. The client is taught to analyze what is being avoided when he or she is anxious and to construct immediately a scene involving the avoided cues or the worst possible outcome of a given situation. By repeating the scene a number of times, while trying to elicit as much anxiety as possible, the client is taught to master "new" fears. *In vivo* exposure is also frequently prescribed for homework. For example, the agoraphobic contracts to venture a specified distance from home each day; the compulsive handwasher agrees not to wash his or her hands more than a specified number of times daily. Such real life exposure is often critical and is described furthur at the end of this chapter.

Anxiety Reduction. The therapist must be aware that some clients will experience a temporary increase in emotional distress prior to improvement (inverted U-shaped extinction function, see p. 31). In such cases, it is assumed that prior to implosive treatment, the client's defensive internal and external avoidance responses (symptoms) have prevented much of the conditioned stimulus complex from eliciting emotion. Presentation of an implosive scene effectively breaks through some of these defenses, exposing more of the stimulus complex and resulting in greater subjective distress. If clients are alerted to this possibility, they are better able to tolerate the distress and to continue with the scenes necessary to reduce the anxiety. Many clients exhibit monotonic reductions in emotion as a function of the amount of exposure to conditioned stimuli. In fact, some clients experience considerable relief and amelioration of symptomatology following a single session. It is preferable, however, to err by needlessly warning these clients of increased distress than to fail to warn those who subsequently show an inverted U-shaped extinction function.

Occasionally, with very well defended clients, little affect is apparent during initial therapy sessions. However, if the therapist is reasonably convinced that the material being presented is relevant, he or she should persevere. Although in theory anxiety activation is necessary for its extinction, research previously reviewed has not as yet supported that position. What has been suggested is that repetition of relevant fear cues is associated with symptomatic improvement. Generally, if the therapist is persistent, emotion will eventually become evident.

Use of Implosive Therapy with Other Therapies

Clients are seen in implosive therapy until their anxiety and anxiety-motivated symptoms decline to their and the therapist's satisfaction. Since implosive therapy may reduce negative emotional response but does not address itself to teaching new behaviors, some clients may benefit from exposure to additional treatment modalities following the implosive sessions. The use of a rational-emotive approach is frequently helpful (Ellis, 1962). Clients may be instructed to assess their "irrational" belief system in an effort to help develop new responses to replace those that were extinguished and to prevent the formation of other avoidance responses as a result of reconditioning to these anxieties and negative affects. When this is done, the client learns both to extinguish the specific avoidance behaviors and to discontinue those behaviors or beliefs that encouraged the development and maintenance of the avoidance behavior. Of course, for some clients such special programs as family therapy, operant retraining programs, or sexual counseling may be beneficial.

Scene Content Areas

Stampfl and Levis (1967) defined 10 areas that "for didactic purposes" are descriptive of common hypothesized cues or stimulus scenes used by the implosive therapist. These include aggression, punishment, oral material, anal material, sexual material, rejection, bodily injury, loss of control, acceptance of conscience, and autonomic and somatic nervous system reactivity. In later writings, they appear to have added an eleventh area which they called inferiority feelings. Brief descriptions of the Stampfl and Levis scene content areas represented didactically follow:

AGGRESSION. Scenes presented in this area usually center around the expression of anger, hostility, and aggression by patient's toward parental, sibling, spouse, or other significant figures in their lives. Various degrees of bodily injury are described, including complete body mutilation and death of the victim.

PUNISHMENT. Patients are instructed to visualize themselves as the recipient of the anger, hostility, and aggression of the various significant individuals in their lives. The punishment inflicted in the scene is frequently a result of the patient's engaging in some forbidden act.

ORAL MATERIAL. In this category oral incorporative and destructive scenes involving, for example, eating, biting, spitting, cannibalism, and sucking are introduced.

ANAL MATERIAL. Anal retentive and expulsive scenes comprising a variety of excretory and related anal situations are described.

SEXUAL MATERIAL. In this area a wide variety of hypothesized cues related to sex are presented. For example, primal and Oedipal scenes as well as scenes of castration, fellatio, and homosexuality are presented.

REJECTION. Scenes where the patient is rejected, deprived, abandoned, shamed, or left helpless are enacted.

BODILY INJURY. Scenes involving mutilation and death of the patient are introduced where fear of injury appears dominant (e.g., in phobic reactions such as falling off a high building, being hit by a car, dying from an infection). This procedure is followed also in cases where suicidal fantasies are present.

LOSS OF CONTROL. Scenes are presented in which patients are encouraged to imagine themselves losing impulse control to such an extent that they act out avoided sexual or aggressive impulses. These scenes usually are followed by scenes where they are directed to visualize themselves hospitalized for the rest of their lives in a back ward of a mental hospital as a result of their loss of impulse control. This area is tapped primarily with patients who express fear of "becoming insane" or concern about being hopeless and incurable.

ACCEPTANCE OF CONSCIENCE. Scenes are portrayed in which the patient confesses, admits, and believes that he or she is responsible and guilty for all sins and wrongdoings (as portrayed in scenes from other categories) through his or her life. The surroundings may be described as involving a courtroom scene with all the patient's family and loved ones present. After the confession, he or she is convicted by the court, sentenced to death, and executed. In some cases, after death the patient is instructed to picture himself going before God where the theme is essentially repeated with God condemning him or her to eternal suffering. An attempt is then made to fit the patient's "hell" to his or her "sins."

ANS AND CNS REACTIVITY. The sensory consequences of autonomic and central nervous system reactivity may themselves function as cues for anxiety. Scenes are introduced in which patients are asked to visualize the sensory consequences of their own nervous system (e.g., heart pounding, perspiration increase, increase in muscular tension, involuntary discharge of the bladder or bowels).

INFERIORITY FEELINGS. Inferiority feelings are described as feelings of inadequacy, cowardice, being a failure, lack of physical beauty or physical strength and abilities. The patient is pictured as a completely inferior person who has "zero" personality resources.

These didactic areas are not intended to be exhaustive of scene content, but they are frequent areas of conflict for many clients. Hence, they may be helpful to the therapist by providing him with areas to examine for hypothesized cues after the symptom-contingent cues have been presented. Scene content for any particular session would not necessarily be restricted to any area, but might cut across the various areas in order to maintain logic and coherence.

Sample implosive scenes within each of the Stampfl–Levis didactic scene content areas are demonstrated in the next section. These scenes or themes are ones that have been used with actual patients. Throughout the scenes, the reasons for using a particular technique is explained. Further detailed case studies of various clinical disorders are presented in Chapter 5.

Sample Transcripts of Scene Content Areas. Implosive therapy and flooding techniques are especially useful with patients who find it difficult to express aggression or feelings of negative affect toward the husband, father, mother, and other men or women in their environment. Lazarus (1971, p. 98) also notes that "when desensitizing patients to 'angry memories'. . .it is usually best to avoid relaxation and similar passive procedures, but instead to have patients picture themselves attacking the offending person." The following case demonstrates the use of implosive therapy with such a person who also suffered from a severe obsessive-compulsive disorder and obsessional fears.

Mrs. J. was a 42-year-old woman who had been married three times, divorced twice, and widowed from her third husband. Her primary problems were difficulty expressing herself and the use of obsessive-compulsive behaviors as avoidance responses for her feelings. She had restricted her life considerably, had been seeing an analyst and, when the therapist first saw her on referral, was confining herself to her apartment. She had given the care of her children over to her parents and was demonstrating a marked withdrawal from all phases of her life. It appeared that her marital problems had stemmed from her lack of assertiveness—she was unable to express her feelings and would withdraw and become passive or passive-aggressive in her response to men. Her unassertiveness seemed to stem from an early hostility toward her father; consequently, the following scene was used to focus on her feelings toward her father. The scene demonstrates the use of such scene content categories as: aggression, punishment, rejection, bodily injury, loss of control, and ANS and CNS reactivity.

I want you to close your eyes and imagine; I want you to visualize as clearly as possible and to act as if you are really there. Imagine that you are at home. It's in the early afternoon sometime in the past; you're alone. I want you to see, to visualize as distinctly as possible the living room of your parent's home. You're sitting there all alone. You can feel the couch, you can see the other chairs, the furniture in the room; it's just starting to get dark. You can see the lights coming on in other houses as you look out the front window. Can you see this now? Visualize it clearly—imagine that you are really there. Try to imagine the smells of your house. You get up and walk across the floor and you can feel the floor pushing up against your feet as you walk along. You walk over to the front door to the house. Put your hand on the door knob, feel the cool knob. Turn the door knob and open the door slowly. Feel the door move out and the fresh air, cool night breeze, early evening breeze comes in and blows across your face. You look out in anticipation of your father coming home. You want to tell him about some of the things that have happened to you today. You are very proud of the fact that you have done well in school. You were elected to a school office, secretary of your class, and you want to tell him about it, even though you are somewhat fearful or anxious that he may not listen to you—he may not praise you—he may not consider the accomplishment worthwhile. After all, he does not seem to feel that you should accomplish these kinds of things. These thoughts are going through your mind now: both pride in yourself and anticipation of your father's response. Can you feel all that? That's fine. See it clearly now. In the driveway you can see your father's car—he comes in through the door and looks at you; he greets you; you run up to give him a hug but he kind of holds back—he never did like you to kiss him or touch him—he kind of pulls back from you and you start to tell him about the day. You tell him about being chosen to be secretary of your class. His response is typical; see him now; he kind of frowns. Look at his face. Look at his face.

It is vital to incorporate facial expressions during scenes using interpersonal situations. Facial expressions are frequently conditioned as cues to oncoming anxiety-provoking scenes. When a patient sees someone's face or facial expression, he or she responds by avoidance. Do not let clients avoid in imagination; encourage them to look at faces. Whenever faces evoke an emotional response, make the client focus on those faces.

See his face; see your father's face; see it clearly now. He starts to frown and he gets that expression that is very familiar to you whenever you try to please him; he is just not pleased—not pleased at all. He feels that you, a young lady, should not be aspiring to do these kinds of things. He thinks you should learn to sew and to cook and to become a good wife and mother, and when he hears your ambitions to go into the business world and become an individual, he finds them not in keeping with his way of thinking. He's very hostile toward these things and you can see that; when you tell him you have actually been elected a class officer, he is not pleased and he makes a very cutting remark. He says, "I suppose this means that you are not going to have time for your home economics course; you are not going to have time to learn those things that are important for a young lady to learn." So you feel hurt and you feel angry. Look at his face; he shakes his head back and forth. In fact, he says, "I don't think I will permit you to be secretary; I don't think you should be doing things like that and I'm going to see if we can't give that position to some young man."

This scene is fairly specific to one situation including symptom-contingent cues and reportable hypothesized cues, but you can probably visualize how the therapist can generalize. This was an actual case and a particular instance in the client's early life when her father had rejected some of her efforts to become independent and respected by her peers.

At this point in the scene presentation, the therapist begins to leave reality and become involved in some of the fantasies that the client must have had as a child.

Now you feel the anger just overwhelming you; it starts to overwhelm you and you start to feel anxious because you are so angry when you look at his face. Feel that anger now? Okay, fine, zero in on it, tune in on it. Feel the hostility and the tension; feel the warmth and the flushing in your face; your hands start to feel cold and you want to scream; you do scream. You turn around and you scream at him. What do you say? What do you say? What do you tell him? Go ahead—you can do it—you tell him.

At this point, the patient indicated some of her feelings about her father's lack of response to her. The therapist should encourage such verbalizations.

That's right; that's what you tell him. You tell him that you really don't appreciate his attitude; not only that but you feel very strongly, very strongly about his attitude and that if he continues, you will probably leave home. He tells you, "No, no you won't—no, you won't leave home." And he takes you by the hand and walks you upstairs; up to your room. Feel him pulling on you, pulling at you, pulling you up those stairs step by step and you are pulling against him yelling, "No, no", and he takes you up to your room and he locks you in your room and he says, "You can come out when you start to act more like a young lady." As you sit there in that room, you feel the hate, yes, the *hate* that you have for him; feel it now, feel it now. You are really angry at him and you are going to plot what you are going to do to him; what you're going to do to get even with him. You are really going to get him. Now, you go over to the closet.

You go over to the closet now; you feel that anger; you feel that anger; let it go. You get yourself a baseball bat; that's right, you get the baseball bat that you've been saving. Feel it in your hands. Feel that bat. I want you to go over to the door; see yourself walking over to your bedroom door. You start pounding on the door with the bat and you beat the door down. You are furious. You are so angry. You beat the door down with the baseball bat and you go downstairs. You see your father sitting there in his chair smoking; see him sitting there so complacently, so smug. Oh, you feel the anger, look at his face; look at that smug face. You know what you'll do with the baseball bat. You know what you're going to do with that baseball bat. Now, what are you going to do?

This technique is called *priming*. In priming, the patient is worked up to a point where he or she can start to express his or her own feelings; the therapist attempts to get the client to supply part of the scene by expressing how he or she would react in the fantasy. The scene is much more realistic if the therapist can get the client involved. In this scene the client might say something like, "I know what I'm going to do; I'm going to hit him." The therapist then coaxes the client along with the scene. If the client does not cooperate then the therapist should continue to direct the scene.

> That's right. You're going to smack him with that baseball bat; you're going to hit him; you're going to *kill* him. (*pause*) You can't stand him; he makes you so angry, so angry and you go over and when he's not looking—he can't see you—you smash him right in the back of the head. You look as he slumps over in the chair; he slumps over in the chair; and he falls and the blood gushes out of his head but you still can't control yourself. The anger is more intense than ever, and you swing that bat and you smash him again on the head and you beat him again and again on the back. You roll him over and you hit him in the stomach; he's barely gasping; barely, just barely breathing. Feel that. See the blood; see it splattered all over everywhere. You have finally done it; you have killed him.

This scene would continue as long as the patient responded. In this particular scene, repetition might be accomplished by having the father not die so soon, but just keep smiling smugly as the client imagines repeatedly beating him and yelling her hate at him. Alternatively, the scene can just be repeated.

> Okay, let's back up, imagine your father telling you, "no, you can't be the secretary"; you will do what *he* wants, not what you wish. See his face, he's stern and angry and somewhat smug in his power and complete control of you—you start to feel the anger.

This same kind of scene could also be repeated with other significant people—particularly significant males, for this client. The point is to help clients respond to those fantasies that they had in the past and are now avoiding because they are too anxiety provoking. Fantasies of a child or younger person are much more objective and straightforward, and when these fantasies recur later in life, we remember how we felt, the tremendous anger and rage that we had. It frightens us; it makes us anxious. Therefore, when the client goes through the fantasy scene, the therapist tells him or her that it is okay to do so; and, in fact, should praise the client for having the courage to go through the fantasy. The client should be encouraged to fantasize on his or her own, to continue until diminution of the emotional response.

A natural progression of this scene would be to go into a punishment scene. With this particular client, the scene was presented as follows:

> Okay, you're standing there; now see yourself standing there looking down at this broken, beaten, battered man. You have totally destroyed him. He is bloody from head to foot; you have beaten all parts of him—his head, his neck, his

shoulders and arms are all maimed and bloody. You continue beating him and you beat his chest, stomach, legs, genitals—all of them totally destroyed. You stand there and look down on this totally mutilated man. Then someone enters the room. Someone comes into the room as you stand there with that bloody baseball bat. See—who is it?

Here again the therapist is priming, asking the client to supply part of the fantasy. The nice thing about implosive therapy is that, if the client comes up with an inappropriate response, the therapist can redirect the fantasy and supply the name of whoever would be most significant, generally either the other parent or a policeman.

You are really afraid that this person is going to come in and see this scene and sure enough, this person enters. Who is it? Who are you afraid will see you now? (*Client responds*)

Your mother, that's right. See her horrified look; her horrified look at you. "What have your done; have you gone *crazy*? How could you possibly have done this—you've gone totally crazy—you've *completely* lost control, you've actually killed your father! You've killed your father." Your mother goes to the phone and calls the police. You just can't move; you just can't believe what you've done and you just stand there and the guilt and the fear and the anxiety overwhelm you. What's going to happen now; what will happen to you?

The rest of the scene could evolve anywhere, but should be consistent with the patient's background. It could involve a combination of loss of control, punishment, and rejection. A typical scene follows.

Okay, now you've done it; you've finally done it! You've totally lost control; you have gone totally out of your mind. The police come in and you see them now. See those tall policemen with boots and they come over and they grab your arm and they put a straitjacket on you and they look at you with horror and disbelief as if there's something basically wrong with you; as if you are something that shouldn't even be touched; and they drag you out to the police car. They drive you to the jail and take you down in the basement and put you in a jail cell.

If the client has an excessive concern over "going crazy," he or she can be taken to the back wards of a mental hospital rather than to a jail cell.

They put you in a jail cell all alone and far removed from anyone else. You feel it now; *you are all alone.* (*pause*)

At this point, the therapist can present scenes of rejection and feelings of loneliness. This is an important area, particularly for clients who have trouble with assertiveness; unassertiveness generally stems from fear of rejection and fear of being alone. The loneliness feelings to portray are basic, described by words like cold, damp, dark, because these terms represent rejection; even the child's early experiences of not having his needs met can be described by these terms.

> Imagine yourself in this jail cell. It's cold . . . dark . . . damp. You are all alone. You can't hear anything. They put you in the back cell like a caged animal; that's what they must think of you. No one is there; no one can see you or hear you and you can see or hear no one else. You are all alone. You have no friends at all. After everybody found out what you did, no one wants to come near you. You are crazy, and you are going to be sorry for what you did. They'll punish you; they'll punish you. They certainly will, and you deserve it; *you killed your own father.*

The scene can develop into a court scene or any place where punishment and cold justice is given out. The therapist should use all the stimulus value of authority to place the punishment on the client. The scene might be a courtroom where the client is down below and the judge sits up very high, a stern father figure.

> You can see him up there, look at his face. Look at the judge's face as he looks down at you. He looks stern at you; he is disgusted by you, and he says, "You are despicable, you are loathsome, you are a horrible person! Look what you did—you killed your father. How could anyone but an animal do what you did. You are not fit to look at!" Everybody is there in the court room—your family, your friends, your relatives. They're all there and they're looking at you and agreeing with the judge. Look back, you can see them standing there now; all shaking their heads in agreement, everyone of them. They think you are a contemptible person.

At this point, the therapist can specifically emphasize the rejection of each individual who is important to the client. The therapist can present vignettes, going through each significant other with the patient—parents (in this case, you've already killed Dad off), spouse, relatives, friends, and presenting each one as rejecting the client because he or she is sinful or because of what he or she has done. In clients who are afraid of loss of affection or are afraid of rejection, this type of scene brings out a tremendous response. Unfortunately, many individuals have spent their lives afraid to stick up for their rights because they fear they would be rejected if they did so. Some clients may have learned this response very early in life and the therapist can work with general scenes as well as specific scenes depicting rejection by parents and special friends. With each scene, the therapist should remind the client that the rejection is based on the client's lack of consideration for that particular person. The final punishment should be whatever is most abhorrent to the client, death in the electric chair, wasting away in a prison cell, or whatever horrible punishment seems applicable to the patient. The therapist can even present scenes following death. Even if the client is not particularly religious, the presentation of a death scene is very important because it represents a basic fear common to most everyone. A scene that is commonly used after death is the fear of being underground. The following scene exemplifies this and is similar to one of Stampfl's favorite scenes.

Imagine that you die but you are still conscious, you are still awake and you realize that you are now going to your own funeral. Imagine that you are in the hearse and you are riding along. You can feel the hearse as it bumps along; feel it. Not one of your friends is there—just you, the hearse driver, and the assistant to help unload the coffin. And you're riding along in a hearse. They are going to put you in the ground somewhere. You can see that you are in a coffin of some kind and you try to get the lid open but you can't move; you are aware of everything but you can't move. You are tied down or so it seems, and you feel the coffin bumping along. Then the hearse stops and you hear the driver and helper talking. They open the door and slide you out of the rear of the hearse; roll you over; jar you around, and the next thing you know you are being lowered slowly down into the ground with vault chains. There is no ceremony—no priest, no family, no friends. You are just being put in the ground; lowering you down, down, down. And then bump! You hit the bottom—feel that. Feel yourself in the bottom of the grave. It's getting colder and it's dark. You start to hear now the sound of the dirt as they throw it in the grave on top of the coffin a shovelful at a time. The dirt hits the casket and it gets darker and darker, colder and colder, and finally all of the light that comes in has been blocked out because you are being covered up—literally buried, buried; dead but aware of everything that is happening. And you feel colder and colder and you are alone and you are dead. Nobody cares. That's the point, you see—you are dead and nobody cares; nobody even cares that you are dead. Then the next thing that you hear is the sound of worms and maggots starting to eat into the coffin; they are going to devour the coffin and then they will devour you. Slowly, you become a stinking, rotten piece of meat. You just deteriorate into the soil and life fades and fades.

Many clients fear that no one loves them, that they will die and no one will care, and that their lives will have been in vain. Thus, they risk all to maintain love, attention, and affection. This scene is useful in helping clients overcome their fear of rejection, fear of loss of love, and fear of being alone. If the client is religious, the therapist can continue the combination punishment–rejection scene in hell. Alternatively, the therapist can present this or similar scenes repeatedly by bringing the client back to life between scenes until the anxiety response to the scene is extinguished. This is a typical scene, but the therapist must make certain that each scene is relevant to the problems of a particular client; if a client does not respond to a scene, the therapist should work through scenes in another manner or move on to another area.

Another obsessive-compulsive patient had a great deal of fear of loss of control and fear of bodily injury. These themes seem to be central to many obsessive-compulsive clients. This particular woman had many rituals that she used to maintain herself. She lived alone and was extremely concerned about keeping everything neat, orderly, and in its proper place. Her compulsiveness prevented her from touching or moving anything. Other fears associated with her fear of not keeping everything in its place were basically due to fear of bodily injury. For example, she was afraid to use the dishes because she was afraid that she might drop and break them and the glass would fly up and cut her. That was her rationale for keeping all of the dishes nicely in place; she used paper plates that she "could throw away easier than she could wash dishes." One of the scenes presented to this client went like this:

> I want you to imagine now, see it clearly. You are standing in the middle of your apartment and you are looking around. You are feeling anxious because there are some things out of place and you are getting more and more anxious *and* at the same time you are just starting to get angry.

This is also priming. Clients who have problems expressing anger toward others can usually respond to the cue to getting angry "at themselves." This anger can then be focused outward.

> You are angry at yourself because you can't live with any uncertainty—you can't live with anything out of place. See your apartment now; see it clearly. The furniture; feel it; the smells of your apartment; see and smell it, it's all there. You notice a plate that is out of place; you had missed it. Now I want you to go over and pick up this plate that has been out of place. You pick it up and just as you pick it up, you realize that it's kind of greasy; it's kind of greasy and slippery. See it; hold it, hold the plate and it starts to slip out of your hand. And it slips slowly; you try to grab it, and it slips, it's going to slip; it's going to fall; feel it slipping slowly out of your hand.

Another important technique is to take the time to describe significant situations in sharp detail. For example, during a scene of aggression, it is frequently important to slow down and have the client *slowly* imagine cutting the body, noticing all of the CS cues that are available, for example, the resistance of the skin, the splitting of the skin, the blood. Similarly, in a death scene when the client is presented as hanging, time should be slowed down and each moment expanded. The feel of the rope around the neck slowly, slowly tightening, the gradual loss of breath, the eventual death should be described. Similarly, this client's fear of losing control of the plate can best be presented in a scene in which it occurs slowly.

> Feel it slowly slipping out of your hand and you grab for it but it's like it has a mind of its own; it's pulling away from you; slipping out of your hands; and it's going to fall. You can feel it; it's going to fall and break into a million pieces, shatter. And all the pieces of glass are going to fly up and hit you and cut you. Feel it now—here it comes! There the plate goes; it's dropping, dropping, and CRASH! (*slaps the desk*) It hit the floor. It is shattering into a million, tiny, sharp pieces of glass. Feel it coming up at you now. Feel the plate; pieces of the plate flying up and cutting you. It's as if an explosion has occurred. Glass is flying up and cutting you all over—cutting your face, your neck, your arms, legs, hands. Feel it now; see the blood start to come—tiny, sharp pieces of glass embedded in your skin. Feel the pain; feel the pain and see the blood.

Pain is a difficult concept to remember and to relate. Therefore, it is important for the therapist to emphasize the conditioned stimuli of blood—the jagged edges of the plate, the look of the cut, the redness of the blood, the blood dripping, and other concrete stimuli associated with the experience of pain.

Sexual material, of course, must be idiographic. There are a number of ways that the therapist can present these scenes but one effective way is to incorporate an age regression aspect. For clients with tensions or anxieties about sexual function, the therapist can begin by presenting a bedroom scene between a man and woman or an actual sexual experience that the client has had. A typical scene presented to a male client follows:

> Imagine that you are in bed, having a sexual experience with your wife; imagine that; feel it now; feel the warmth, the pleasant sensations as you each stroke the other's body. You feel the sensation in your groin. Feel your penis becoming erect; it's getting hard; you're starting to enjoy the sensations and you begin to become more involved. You start to reach out to your partner, your wife. What do you hear? Look over your shoulder and there—you don't know how she got there, but there she is—looking into your bedroom door. There's your mother. See her face. See the disapproving, shocked, stern expression on her face. Feel your penis go limp.

This would be an initial scene. Masturbatory scenes, depicting earlier experiences in which the patient was punished for sexual activity would follow. These sexual scenes, especially early masturbatory scenes, are very effective for patients who are sexually inhibited and have problems expressing themselves sexually.

Acceptance of conscience is an important theme. During scenes of rejection, aggression, counter-aggression, and punishment, the therapist may emphasize that the client "really is sinful and guilty." The therapist denies any statements that the client is being persecuted and impresses upon the client that he deserves rejection and punishment. The acceptance of conscience scene that is presented below was used with the previously discussed nonassertive woman (Mrs. J.):

> You see your mother; she is looking at you and she yells at you, "You are no good. You totally lost control and you killed your father." You agree with her; you know that you deserve this punishment. "You are really rotten and despicable. How could anybody do what you did? You must be ruthless; you are so sinful that you have no rights; you cannot be forgiven. No one could possibly forgive such an atrocious act. You've always been like this; you've always had these thoughts, these terrible hideous thoughts. You've always been guilty; you really are guilty. You really are a horrible person." Feel that now.

Physiological sensations occur throughout scene presentation and it is important for the client to focus on these bodily reactions. The therapist should remind the client to zero in on those types of feelings that are considered anxiety-provoking. Prior to beginning scene presentation, the client should be instructed, when the therapist asks, "What do you feel?" to report physiological sensations (e.g., "tight in my chest" or "my throat is dry") and "gut reactions" to the particular scene, not psychological interpretation such as "I feel guilty or anxious." By knowing the client's particular physiological response to anxiety cues from earlier inquiry, the therapist can prompt these reactions.

> Feel it now, concentrate on it. You are upset; your hands are cold and clammy; your hands are perspiring. Your stomach feels upset and you feel nauseous. Feel it now. It's going to get worse. Make it worse.

Finally, we have not emphasized the dynamic areas of anal, oral, or phallic material. However, if they are deemed significant, the use of primal scenes, early fears of being rejected, cold and unfed as a child and baby (pulled away from the breast), castration fears, and punishment might be appropriate; scenes related to early loss of control problems such as bed wetting, and throwing of temper tantrums might be used if they are effective in eliciting anxiety.

The Flooding Technique

Imaginal Flooding

We have already discussed the issue of distinguishing between flooding and implosive therapy. From a clinical standpoint the distinction is even harder to discern. Imaginal flooding is basically the practice of limiting exposure content to symptom-contingent cues only. Implosive therapists generally include hypothesized material. From a clinical standpoint then, the distinction between flooding and implosive therapy blurs into a continuum of session content, with concrete material (i.e., symptom-contingent cues) at one end and abstract hypothesized cues (i.e., psychodynamic scenes) at the other. In our own practice, we use almost all levels of the continuum, depending on the patient response.

Thus, having a separate section of the imaginal flooding vis-à-vis implosive therapy is not easily integrated into our perception of exposure methodology, but rather, such a separation is forced by the semantics of the literature. We have already discussed what amounts to imaginal flooding in the section on implosive therapy.

In Vivo Flooding

In vivo flooding has been shown to be an extremely effective treatment for agoraphobia, specific phobias, and compulsive disorders. Much of the research on *in vivo* exposure has involved the therapist accompanying a client or a group of clients into the feared environment. There are, however, several practical disadvantages to using *in vivo* flooding where the therapist directs the sessions in person. First of all, it is time-consuming and expensive. Therapist directed *in vivo* flooding may require travel to the feared stimulus or environment. Second, since long sessions of up to three hours are most effective, one patient could make the scheduling difficult for a busy therapist with a variety of commitments. Third, the average clinician may not see enough patients with problems that are treatable by *in vivo* exposure to develop groups. Finally, *in vivo* exposure may require the therapist to perform onerous tasks for which they are not trained or at least not interested in performing. For example, one of us has treated several cockroach phobics. Trapping and maintaining live cockroaches is not enjoyable.

On the other hand, it is possible to contract with clients to carry out *in vivo* exposure successfully on their own (Mathews *et al.*, 1977; Emmelkamp, 1974; Griest *et al.*, 1980). In our practice, we often demonstrate *in vivo* flooding by having a therapist directed session using both *in vivo* and imaginal flooding (e.g., a trip to the store with the therapist; a short drive in traffic with the therapist) in which specific procedures are demonstrated allowing the client to then carry out the therapy task as homework. When a contract for *in vivo* homework is made, the therapist should be very specific as to the exact behavior being contracted for, the time of day it should be carried out, and the number of times per day or week that the client is required to engage in the behavior. Phobic clients have a strong tendency to avoid, and are ingenious at coming up with "good reasons" for excusing themselves from homework. Being very specific about the terms of the contract and emphasizing the importance of doing the homework reduces resistance. Another advantage of homework over therapist directed *in vivo* exposure is that many phobics experience fear in the presence of the phobic object or situation only when they are alone. Often driving phobics, for example, will never experience fear when the therapist is with them.

Finally, the "gradedness" of *in vivo* flooding must be carefully evaluated. If clients are required to engage in behavior that immediately brings on a full-blown panic attack, there is a good chance that they will not continue with the homework. Further, many clients simply refuse to start out in the most fearful situation. In general, we emphasize two things to the client: (1) the importance of "going as far as possible" and (2) never leaving the feared situation or object in a panic, but rather waiting, if at all possible, until the panic state subsides before departing. We stress to the client that, from our theoretical view, fleeing the feared situation in a panic defeats any gains that may have been made and may even increase the symptomatic avoidance behavior through operant conditioning.

There is one form of therapist-directed *in vivo* exposure that does not have any of the practical disadvantages previously mentioned. This involves having the client or significant other bring phobic objects into the therapy session. For example, "contaminated" objects can be brought in a plastic bag. One woman, for instance, unable to enter a "contaminated" room in her house, brought in much of the furniture piecemeal.

In summary, *in vivo* flooding is an effective technique for treating fears and obsessive-compulsive disorders. There are, however, several practical disadvantages for the average therapist who wishes to use therapist-directed *in vivo* flooding. When possible, contracting with the client to carry out *in vivo* homework assignments, or to bring phobic objects into the therapy session, may be just as effective and have fewer practical disadvantages. *In vivo* flooding, as used with a variety of disorders, is discussed and demonstrated with the case material in Chapter 5.

5

CASE EXAMPLES

Most anxiety-based disorders can be effectively treated with flooding and/or implosive therapy. In this chapter, we describe flooding and implosive therapy as they are used in our clinical practice. Several disorders are discussed and appropriate case studies are presented. We, of course, cannot describe treatment for all the specific disorders for which exposure is appropriate. The cases selected are representative of the types of clients and disorders that respond well to this treatment. Where we felt it would be helpful, transcripts of implosive and flooding scenes are presented. Further, even though the more complex anxiety disorder of agoraphobia and perhaps many obsessive-compulsive disorders are best treated in groups, we have chosen to present only cases treated individually. Most therapists do not see enough clients to form groups for these complex disorders. Chambless and Goldstein (1981) offer an excellent description of an effective group treatment program using exposure techniques.

In reading this chapter, it will become obvious that flooding and implosive therapy are not the only things we do with clients. Behavior therapists are often described as having "tunnel vision"; that is, applying their techniques across the board without asking for feedback from the client and without concern for how the client feels or what and how he or she thinks. Professionals who have an active practice know that such an attitude not only leads to ineffective treatment but also results in the loss of clientele.

In implosive therapy it is often necessary to present scenes that would normally appear to the layman as terrifying, disgusting, or otherwise aversive. Because the purpose of this chapter is to demonstrate exposure therapy, the scene content itself is emphasized in the case examples that follow. Again, we wish to point out, however, that when the therapist is not presenting implosive or flooding scenes, it is vitally important that he or she convey empathy and support to the patient. The maintenance of a supportive client–therapist relationship is crucial to the success of any therapy and perhaps even more so to a treatment that requires clients to experience anxiety or other conditioned emotional responses that they would normally prefer to avoid. As we have already emphasized, exposure techniques have been shown to be effective, and there is no evidence that implosive therapy and/or flooding is dangerous or produces negative side affects. The bottom line is that this psychological treatment may not always be pleasant, but it works; an analysis that could be applied to many medical or surgical treatments as well.

DSM-III describes six anxiety disorders that we feel can be effectively treated with exposure: (1) chronic posttraumatic stress, (2) simple phobias; (3) social phobia; (4) agoraphobia; (5) panic disorders; and (6) obsessive-compulsive disorders. What follows are case examples of clients suffering from these disorders who were treated by one or the other of us, with some form of exposure therapy. This first case is the only example in this chapter in which an extensive portion of the diagnostic interview is transcripted. We feel this interview is quite typical of the type of diagnostic interview we use for implosive-therapy clients.

Chronic Posttraumatic Stress Disorder

Posttraumatic stress disorder involves the unwanted reexperiencing of a traumatic event. Often the stressful incidence occurs in the form of dreams. With some individuals, the anxiety originally associated with the traumatic event may be experienced when they are in the presence of a stimulus that is similar to that which set off the original trauma. Thus, some veterans of wars are overly sensitive to sudden loud noises that set off autonomic or cognitive symptoms similar to those experienced in the war. Some individuals who suffer from this disorder experience intensive thoughts and/or fugue states in which they may relive the experience for an extended period of time. Clients may complain of feeling estranged from people, a flattening of affect, and the inability to express positive emotions. Guilt about surviving when friends have died or over heinous acts committed in war may be present. Anger, hostility, and aggressiveness, as well as the use of drugs or alcohol, are common coping mechanisms.

Individuals who suffer from negative emotions that have their origin in severe trauma(s) generally respond well to implosive or flooding therapy. Both of the authors have worked in VA hospitals and have treated many cases of posttraumatic stress disorder that originated during combat (war neurosis). The following cases are interesting and typical exmaples of postraumatic stress disorder that were successfully treated with implosive therapy. The first case presented includes a transcript of a clinical interview that was conducted prior to treatment. Although this interview is with a patient suffering from postraumatic stress, it exemplifies the type of information needed by any therapist anticipating using implosive therapy or flooding. As such, it is a general example of the type of interview we conduct with all patients.

Case Study

George, a 26-year-old Vietnam war veteran at the time of treatment, complained of what he called a thunderstorm phobia. He stated that he could not continue to work or stay outside during a thunderstorm or when one was predicted. Because of this, he had lost several outside jobs. George was also sensitive to sudden loud noises. He stated that he felt obsessed with his fear because he felt it necessary to listen for weather reports and watch the sky constantly. When a storm was imminent, or when he heard the first rumbling of thunder, he would go to a basement area. During long storms he would often drink beer to reduce his anxiety. He would sometimes try to "outrun" storms by getting into his car and driving as fast as possible.

George could not remember exactly when he first experiened the storm fear, but was certain that it did not predate his Vietnam experience. He did relate his fear of loud noises to several traumatic experiences while he was in Vietnam. He had on several occasions experienced near misses in which mortar shells and mines were set off close to him, knocking him down and, on one occasion, throwing him 30 feet through the air. The experience that seemed most relevant to him occurred when he was riding a troop carrier in a small patrol mission. On this occasion, George was the last vehicle in the patrol convoy. (A safe place, he noted, if they were to run over mines.) At one point, however, for reasons not altogether clear, the patrol was ordered to reverse the convoy. This maneuver, in effect, placed his carrier at the front of the convoy. Not long after that, George experienced a "crushing wave" that picked him up and threw him through the air. He noted that just before he hit the ground, he felt a "hot" feeling in his chest and heard a very loud exploson. As a result of the explosion, he was knocked unconscious for several minutes.

The troop carrier had hit a land mine. George was the only survivor of that carrier. He sustained several injuries from the impact, most notably a chest wound and several facial contusions and cuts. He later required surgery and plastic surgery to repair the wounds. Even though George had no fear of storms immediately following this event, he still relates the two because during storms he experienced the same hot feeling in his chest and what seemed like a similar surge of air pressure.

George's early life experiences were unremarkable. He grew up in a small town, graduated from high school, and had been drafted and spent four years in the military. After receiving an honorable discharge, he used his GI bill to go to school. His occupational goals were vague but his fantasy goal was to become an actor. He had several long and serious relationships with women but had never married. He noted that his fear of loud noises and thunderstorms had also interfered with his personal life. He felt that having these fears had undermined his self-confidence and made him less effective in his interactions with others. He found it difficult to show true affection for his girlfriend.

His treatment goal was to overcome his fear of storms so that he could consider better occupations and so that he could feel more acceptable to others. He felt that other people would consider anyone who was afraid of thunderstorms as either weak or crazy.

FIRST INTERVIEW

Therapist. You told me that you felt more tense when you were in a storm, especially a thunderstorm but that any loud noise or quick movement would bring on a very tense or anxious feeling in you. Thunderstorms were mentioned as well as wind and rain on the roof. A truck started up one time and that bothered you. When airplanes fly over the house, the noise sometimes brings on anxiety. You said something about the TV and that you were imaging that it might blow up. Can you explain this?

Client. If I am watching TV and it suddenly goes off because of video difficulty, I start imagining something is happening, you know, the quickness.

T. Do you go on and think through this?

C. Actually, I get up and look out the window to see if there is a big flash of lightning and things of this nature.

T. So it's like an expectation you have.

C. Yes.

T. And during this, what do you feel?

C. I feel heat in my chest and a shivering sensation. I get very anxious anticipating what's coming.

T. One of the things I'm interested in for the kind of treatment that we are planning is to find out specifically what these feelings are. You mentioned heat in your chest. You feel like your chest gets warm or hot.

C. It gets exceedingly hot.

T. Is there a tingling sensation along with that?

C. Yes. When the thunderstorm begins, it sets up a tense feeling in me. Thunderstorms are actually the basis of most of my big anxiety attacks because they are more like explosions—the light, the flash, the hitting, and the rumbling of the ground, etc. I keep up with the weather conditions quite well. I anticipate storms and it sort of puts me on edge. I get a tightness in my muscles. I try to go somewhere to get away from the storm, but if I'm in it or if it's right over, then I can feel the heart and the burning sensations that I had in Vietnam.

T. OK. When you say "I had," what you're talking about is some earlier experience. You trace back the response that you have to these kinds of stimuli to some early war experiences that you have had so that the tight feeling, the anticipation, the heat. . .

C. I actually feel the fire.

T. It feels hot like you feel the fire.

C. Yes. It sort of seems to swell up and get more intense.

T. What other kinds of symptoms do you have?

C. It seems that my heart is going to just jump right out of me. It seems to get worse and worse. Then I will start running or I will get in the car and try to go somewhere enclosed where there are no windows or where a lot of people are where I have to act normal.

T. What do people do for you besides make you act normal?

C. Well, they don't do anything for me, I guess, because I don't tell them I'm scared. It might scare somebody and I really don't want anybody to know it. But it makes me socialize, so it makes me act normal and then I'm fighting the anxiety. So I believe, if I can understand it, I can beat it. That's the thing that is the most in my mind right now. I can't seem to control it and understand why it does it because, even when it's happening to me, I know that nothing is wrong, but I still can't control it.

T. Does it ever seem like the tension and anxiety that you feel actually increase the anxiety. . .as if you expect this tenseness and fear to come over you and just knowing that this might happen makes your more anxious?

C. I believe so. . .yes.

T. It kind of feeds on itself then?

C. Yes. Because I have a lack of understanding.

T. You deal with this problem by running to an enclosed place or to a place where people are, where you will have to maintain some composure and perhaps talk with them and socialize to distract you from your anxiety. Are there any other things that you do?

C. If I'm in a car when a storm begins, I will try to outrun it or go around it. I look for the flashes and I try to get away from them—even to the point several times where I almost had a wreck.

T. So you drive fast sometimes?

C. I don't drive fast but I'm wreck-prone. I have just got to get away. I try to drive as carefully as possible, but sometimes it's overwhelming, the heat, the adrenaline pumping, and so forth. I pick safe roads to try to go, but if anybody is in my way, I will go around them. If a light is red, it has no bearing on me whatsoever. I'll stop and make sure no cars are coming, but I'll still go through the redlight.

T. To sum up, there are certain kinds of situations that usually involve some kind of quick movement, a thunderstorm or a loud noise, that can set off this anxiety reaction in you, which is characterized by heat, tingling, and tightness in the chest. You feel the tenseness in your muscles, your heart starts to pound, and you feel like you're starting to shiver. Then you want to run from it.*

C. I want to move. I just want to keep moving. I feel the heat in the back of my head and it seems like it sort of runs up my spine and up my chest.

T. You said, "If I could just understand why?" Let's put that aside for now because, as I have indicated to you, we may never know "why", but we can still work with the problem. We can guess at why, but let's just try now to get some history. When is the first time you felt this happen to you? You can trace it back to some incidences in Vietnam. Could you describe those situations for me now?

C. Well, the main one, I think, that set it off was the fact that I got blown-up. I was on a troop carrier and we were on a mission and hit a mine. It killed everyone else except me. I was the back machine gunner and I was sitting on the back turret. We had just made a reverse march, which was not unusual. The quickness of the explosion was so tremendous, that's the way I feel when something happens. But anyway, when it blew up, it blew up in the front, but all the compression came through the vehicle and got me.

T. And you felt the warmth?

C. Yes. It was fire. I don't remember it except in a flash. That's what really got me was the quickness of it. It was just a BOOM and I landed out in the field somewhere. As I was going through the air, I wasn't conscious, but I guess my subconscious was telling me, "No, don't let it be me." When I hit the ground, I was alive. I was burnt, hurting, and everything.

T. Now tell me everything that you can remember and be as specific as possible. You said you were on some sort of routine mission. What exactly was it?†

C. Well, it was a reconnaissance mission but those missions turn into anything. Actually, what we were doing was just searching that area. We had another platoon with us on top of the vehicle. We had about six or seven vehicles. We had been out there three or four days in a row.

T. Was it night?

C. No, it was in the morning.

T. You had been out in the field for. . .

C. We had been out there three or four days in a row in the same area. We just started going back. I really don't know why we were going back; it was general orders was all we knew.

T. OK. At this point, your tension and anxiety levels were not too high because you were on your way back and you had been there before; you didn't really anticipate this at all.

*It is important to understand the exact sensation (CNS and ANS feedback) so that they may be recreated in the implosive scene.

†Specific details are important to the implosive therapist so that accurate scenes can be presented later.

C. Well, we always anticipate things but nothing like this. It's like being in love, you don't know what it's like until you have actually been there. I had no idea.
T. So you were through with your mission and you were on your way back?
C. No, we were just beginning. What had happened is that we had taken the wrong road. I won't get into that, because there was a lot of chaos about that. We missed the road; we had been down it three or four days before but, for some reason, we missed the road.
T. Whoever was driving missed it?
C. Right. So they called a reverse march which means the back vehicle takes the lead and goes back and that made us the lead vehicle. As luck would have it, we started down the right road and that's when it hit us. It was tremendous. It killed everybody in the crew.
T. Tell me about your crew. Were you close with that crew?
C. I was close to one person in that crew. I tried not to get close to people because I knew in that situation that it just wouldn't be any good to. . .
T. What was his name?
C. I don't remember. I guess I have tried to forget it. Maybe I will remember in a few minutes.
T. Was there one person in this group that you had become friends with that you had known for sometime?
C. Yes, I respected him. He seemed to have his stuff together.
T. Was he above you in rank?
C. Yes. I believe he was. He had been there longer.
T. He wasn't your sergeant or anything like that?
C. No. He was our driver.
T. What was your position and what were you called officially?
C. Machine gunner.
T. Your rank?
C. I think I was an E-3.
T. An E-3 which is like a PFC?
C. Yes.
T. Were you drafted?
C. Yes.
T. Did you want to be in the service?
C. Well, I had two brothers in the Air Force. It didn't matter, actually. I can't remember but I think I put down Vietnam as a choice when I did get drafted; it meant nothing and I knew it.
T. How did you feel about the war? Did you feel that we should have been there?
C. I feel that we should have been there, but I feel like we should have done something. We should have not been held back so much.
T. OK.
C. A lot of people felt that way.
T. How do you feel about it now?
C. I'm not mad or anything like that. I feel like it was sort of a waste—that we wasted all those lives and time and then didn't hold it.

T. OK. You were on a reverse march going back and you had just turned to go onto the right road when you felt this tremendous explosion, flash, and heat. Did you see a flash or what did you see?
C. As if one of those lights burst or a flash of lightning when you don't expect it.
T. And then you felt this impact.
C. Yes. A tremendous impact that threw me about 30 feet.
T. Then you don't remember anything for a while or what?
C. Well, I thought I was dead, to be honest about it.
T. What do you recall? Did you have any kind of dream? Sometimes people have sensations when they are out.
C. Actually, I thought I was dying and I thought, "Oh God, not me, not this time." I actually felt like I was dying. I guess it was the sensation of flying through the air that gave me a floating sensation. When I hit the ground, it sort of knocked me back.
T. A floating *sensation*? But, you did actually fly through the air, didn't you?
C. Yes.
T. While this was happening, you thought, "This is it?"
C. Yes. The impact and the quickness; I just can't explain it. It's like somebody having a ballbat and you not even seeing it and they just go WHAM. I just felt like I was dying. When I hit the ground, my eyes were all blurred. They were burnt. I was burnt from approximately half of the top of my head down, but I knew I was alive. I ran back towards the vehicle or towards the rest of the vehicles and I think I grabbed my TC.
T. Your what?
C. The TC, the man who runs the vehicle. . .the sergeant or whoever and he was burnt. He was a black man and he was burnt completely except for just a couple of little spots. I tried to grab a piece of clothing or whatever. I guess I was in a daze or shock. But then we ran back to the other vehicles, and I think there was shooting going on. I had my 45 out. That's the only thing I had left. I guess I was just acting on habit or impulse. When I got back there, I realized I could hardly see at all.
T. Did you think you were going blind?
C. I had thoughts of, "Please don't make me blind." I hollered for Doc, who was another PFC, and he put some gauze in my eye. I still had the 45 in my hand. The guy in the helicopter asked me if he could have my gun and I said, "I don't know; where are we?" He said I was safe and not to worry.
T. Then you went to. . .
C. The hospital.
T. There weren't any serious injuries? Did they have to do any kind of skin grafting?
C. No, I don't know which is worst, first degree burns or third degree burns, but, whichever is less, then that's what mine were.
T. OK. Then you felt that, after your burns healed, you were OK.?
C. Well, my back was hurt quite a bit. I caught some schrapnel in it and landed on some trees.
T. So they picked some fragments out of your back?

C. I think so. After that, when incoming would come in, I felt that again. I didn't feel the regular "get in the hole and pray" type of thing.
T. When what would come in?
C. Incoming. Incoming shells from the rockets. They would stand about two miles away and shoot them at us.
T. You'd feel this?
C. Yes. I noticed it.
T. You felt the heat?
C. Yes. I felt that again. I relived that situation, not the one that was happening. I didn't want to say anything because, at the time in that situation, they might call you a chicken or something, if you said something was wrong. I thought it, which everybody did then, because incoming was a terrible thing. You didn't know where it was coming from or where it was going to hit. This was linked with the fact that I didn't know that bomb was there. I guess that's the reason I got the same sensations. Then I had a machine gun blowup in my face.
T. Now, are you going into the next incident in Vietnam that you feel might be related to this?
C. The things I feel that are related to it are getting blown up to begin with, then the machine gun blowing up in my face.
T. OK. Tell me about that now.
C. I was firing.
T. Was this after the first incident?
C. Yes.
T. And you were firing your machine gun?
C. We were not on the turret; we were just on the range.
T. Were you practicing or fighting?
C. We were practicing. Actually, it was old ammunition and we would go out and shoot it away.
T. OK. You were doing this and what happened?
C. The bullet jammed and fired in my face and knocked me off the back of the vehicle. It was the same thing all over again. It burnt my face. It was almost a small reenactment of the first time, except I got the full impact of that machine gun right smack in the kisser instead of just a burning.
T. What was the result of that? What did you do then?
C. I'm sorry, I don't understand.
T. What happened then. It knocked you off the vehicle. Where you knocked out?
C. I was almost knocked out. Not completely. My face was burnt. I had powder burns on my face and chest. I just started running around in circles trying to rip my clothes off because I thought I was on fire because I was so hot. I threw my helmet off and went to the jeep where the captain was and asked him if my face was messed up or burned or something like that.
T. Do you remember who your captain was and why did you run to the captain?
C. It was the closest place to run. He was watching us fire. I didn't know who was in the jeep. I don't even know if it was him I talked to. I talked to somebody in a jeep.

T. And you said what?
C. I asked was my faced burned, am I all right, is anything wrong?
T. OK. Were there any problems?
C. There were some small burns but not bad. There were little tiny holes in my face.
T. Did you go to the hospital?
C. They took me to the med-station on the base.
T. Then did they release you?
C. Yes.
T. Then, what was the next incident that you think might be related.
C. Well, I was hit by lightning. I wasn't actually hit by lightning, the building was.
T. The building you were in was hit by lightning?
C. Yes. We were sitting in the building and there was a tremendous storm which was bothering me already. But, like I said, I was doing my best to cope with it because there wasn't anything I could do about it. The anxiety had not grown in intensity at that point; I guess the situation I was in, and where I was at, had something to do with it. I had to deal with it. We were sitting there drinking a few beers and there was a tremendous storm. There was a monsoon with tremedous lightning. It was a bad electrical storm. I think it hit the top of the building and it just knocked me completely across the room and I hit up against a locker. There was a tremendous surge of heat and tightness coming over me. There was a burning sensation.
T. OK. Was there another time?
C. Other than the times of just getting hit by mortar, I guess not. I was in a metal bunker one time; I jumped in it because of incoming. A couple of them landed a few feet away. That echoing brought it on. I just thought it was tremendous fear because the fear was of dying. But I had the same sensation, just like the first incident. It seemed like everything went right back to the first one. After I learned that fear, it seemed everything else brought on that fear and no other.
T. Before you went to Vietnam, did you ever have any problems with tension or anxiety?
C. No. I was the most outgoing character you ever met.
T. You say outgoing. Are you saying that somehow these events have made you less outgoing?
C. I don't know. I think what it is is that I try to foresee something happening and stop it. Like going out to a dance or something. If there is a bad reputation, I won't go. That's just it.
T. What do you mean, "A bad reputation?"
C. Well, something like fights or the people who patronize the place. I don't want to get into those situations.
T. So the potential for violence is something that is anxiety provoking for you? If somebody gets up and starts trouble, what happens to you then?
C. I just get mad, but luckily nothing has ever happened.
T. Do you feel you would strike back then?

C. Yes.
T. Do you think that this might be related to these others?
C. I don't know. I don't think I'm a violent person. I'm not. As a matter of fact, I am exactly the opposite. I will go out of my way not to fight. In other words, I don't want to get into that situation again. I don't want to be hurt again. I have been hurt enough.
T. It makes you anxious, too, especially when you start to feel these sensations?
C. Yes.
T. What other kinds of situations do you avoid?
C. Well, I don't know. They are so numerous. I really don't know off the top of my head. I can't recall. Well, I actually avoid the highway. It scares me. Well, it doesn't scare me, it's just so much going on.
T. OK. You mean the traffic on the expressway.
C. Yes. But what I don't like is that I don't trust them.
T. Are you saying that you don't want to be in situations where people around you might not be trustworthy? In other words, where you might not be sure of what they are going to do, such as getting angry with you, or they might lose control of themselves causing a problem for you?
C. Right.
T. So the guy might get angry at someone else across the room and shoot at him and instead hit you.
C. Right.
T. So it's not so much that these situations are going to get you into trouble but that you don't want to be around anyone who is not in control or may lose control.
C. Well, I think that the bottom line of it is the fact of the quickness of the unknown. I don't know how to say it but like the quickness that something could happen and you can't control it. You don't have any control over it. I try to foresee something before and not put myself into that situation where something could happen so quick that I couldn't do anything about it.
T. Let's go back now. I think I have a good understanding of that. I would like to get a few basic answers. First of all, were you raised by your family?
C. Yes. My father died when I was 8 months old.
T. So your mother raised you. Alone?
C. Yes.
T. Did she ever remarry?
C. She didn't remarry but she has had a boyfriend for about 17 or 18 years.
T. Was he a father figure for you at all?
C. In a great sense, yes.
T. It's important for the therapy that we will be using that I know names of people. Not last names but first names.
C. His name is Joe.
T. OK. He was like a father to you, but was your mother the dominant figure?
C. Right, sure. I felt a great sense of responsibility, even at a young age. I never knew my father or what it is like to have a father, so I don't think I ever really

missed it. Joe was more of a friend than anything else. There is no real closeness.

T. He didn't punish you?

C. No.

T. Did your mother punish you?

C. Every now and then.

T. What was her technique?

C. She would whip me.

T. She would use a whip?

C. Not a whip but she would use what we call a hickory switch.

T. And where would she hit you with that?

C. On the butt. Usually I would get away from her.

T. So that was the main kind of punishment. Did she continue to use that after you got older?

C. No. As a matter of fact, I can't bring to mind any one certain time that I got one.

T. It wasn't a significant thing then? It was just what she used and when she got the hickory stick out you knew that it was time to shape up or get the hell out of there, huh? (*laughs*)

C. Right.

T. You can't recall any specific times when she used the hickory stick when you were young for doing something?

C. No, not really.

T. Did you call her mom?

C. Yes.

T. How would you characterize your mother? Would you say she was strict or lenient?

C. A long time ago, she played ball and did things like that with us. She was a really outgoing mother. She would get right out there with us. But in recent years she has become what I call a hypochondriac.

T. You think she's a hypochondriac?

C. Yes. I think she does have tremendous symptoms of it. That's just my opinion. She always worries about dying of cancer. If somebody gets it, she thinks about it. She has put on a little weight. She has changed a lot... (*Some further discussion here*)

T. How many brothers and sisters do you have?

C. Two brothers.

T. Older or younger?

C. Older.

T. And what are their names?

C. Jack and Harry.

T. Do you call them Jack and Harry?

C. No. I call them Jack and Buddy.

T. What did your father die from?

C. Actually, he died from a man choking him, but he was drowned, I think is the way it is said. They were in a boat fishing and it capsized and he pulled one man to the bank and then went back after the other one and the other one choked him. They both went down.

T. So he was trying to save someone?

C. Yes. The guy was in shock and didn't know what he was holding to and choked him.

T. Did the other man see this happening?

C. I guess so. That's how I got the story.

T. Did you have some reason to believe that might not have been the whole story?

C. No. That's just what my mother told me. I didn't figure she would want to go into any great detail about someone standing on the bank watching.

T. Why do you suppose she never married Joe?

C. Well, she had to work quite a bit with three boys and she didn't have a very good education.

T. But she never married Joe. Do you know why?

C. I don't know. They won't tell me.

T. Did you have any feelings about that?

C. No.

T. But they still live together?

C. No. They don't live together. They live side by side—two houses beside each other. He's one of the guys that never got away from home after the first marriage and he got divorced and had two or three children by his other marriage, so he moved back in with his family. His other brothers lived there, too. Then he bought a house on the other side of the park and we fixed it up and Mom moved in there.

T. OK. Just briefly, have you ever had any thoughts about this? Your father and the way he died. Did you ever dream about it or have early memories? Do you recall ever imagining what went on?

C. Well, not really. I have thought probably what happened was that everybody was out there drinking and having a ball and somebody made a mistake and stood up or something.

T. Sometimes when things like this happen when we are very young, the response of a child when he sees other fathers with their sons is to be kind of angry at his father, even though he knows it wasn't his fault or to, perhaps as you say, "blame" him that he was drinking or something like that and just for an instant feel kind of angry that you don't have a father. Have you ever felt that way?

C. No. That's why I say, I don't know where I got it from but I have always had a responsible attitude.

T. Which of your two older brothers was more like a father to you?

C. Neither. I had to do it myself. We were rousty guys.

T. Did you get into a lot of fights with them?

C. No, not really. We only had one or two that I can remember.

T. Did you bicker a lot when you were kids?

C. Well, they "bickered" on me because I was the smallest but, other than that, no.

T. Did you feel like you were picked on?
C. Yes. Well, I most definitely was every now and then.
T. How about Jack and Buddy? Are they getting along pretty well?
C. No, they don't get along very well.
T. Why not?
C. I don't know. Probably, mainly because of my older brother. He has spent 12 years in the Air Force. He has just had problem after problem and it has made him a not very likeable fellow.
T. What kind of problems has he had?
C. Well, his wife left him after 12 years of marriage. She was a slob, really. When they came back when he was getting ready to get out of service, we went over to their house and they had stuff packed up in corners, walls, and everything. They had been sitting there for two years. Jack is a little like me—kind of a perfectionist. I didn't see how he could live like that. Finally, he lost her and his two kids. He got out of the Air Force but I really don't think he wanted to, but his immediate family pushed him to the point of it. He has had a couple of bad incidences lately, such as getting locked up for drunk driving twice and he can't seem to find a job. He was a technical engineer for 12 years, and now he tells them "technical engineer" in civilian life and they tell him, "You've got to start here" and that really gets to him. I think he's got a fight-against-the-world type of attitude.
T. And Buddy?
C. Buddy is sort of quiet and reserved but conniving. He doesn't seem to care for too much of anything except going fishing.
T. So neither one of them has a job?
C. Yes. They both work.
T. They just don't have the kind of job they *could* have?
C. Yes. They could do better. But you know, that's them. I don't care. The thing that tore them apart is their personalities. They won't even get together and talk.
T. OK., I think that's probably enough for this session. I would like to have one more interview with you. OK.?
C. OK.

Second Interview

T. Last time we went over the symptoms. We talked about the heat in the chest, the tightness of muscles, and the feeling of swelling up; your heart jumps and you stiffen. You mentioned the heat in the back of the head occurring with loud noises, thunderstorms especially, and anything that would be similar to the experiences you had in Vietnam. So we have a good idea of the specific instances which you feel were responsible for some of the problems that you have now. Then we went back and talked a little bit about your family and talked about your two brothers and the fact that your father died when you were young. Today I would like to talk to you about some of the more recent experiences you have had and then, in contrast, some of your very early life experiences and discuss any dreams that you have. I will also ask you to do some exercises so I can see how well you visualize and imagine things, so that I will have an understanding of how to work with you when we get into treatment. Now you mentioned thunderstorms. Can you remember after you got out of Vietnam and you felt that you were still kind of anxious about loud noises and were feeling a little uptight about those kinds of things? I think you told me. "Well, hell, that will go away, I'll get over that."

C. I was told that it would. One of the psychologists told me. I just went in there one day and he sort of said it would go away. So I took it for what it was worth and just tried to do the best I could with it. It sounded reasonable and then I was coming back to not anything like that, so I thought surely it would go away with no problem.

T. Did you then just kind of forget about it?

C. No. I didn't forget about it. It continued, but I thought it would sort of dwindle down.

T. Did you see any change in your response over time?

C. If anything, it worsened. That's the reason I started seeking help. I went through two summers and it seemed to get worse. I seemed to be more withdrawn and then I started looking for somebody to help me.

T. Can you tell me how this problem significantly interferes with your life?

C. Well, it interferes with everything.

T. Can you give me some examples? How, for instance, does it interfere with your ability to work and maintain a job?

C. Well, I don't like to work around loud machinery. If I am at a job, I feel if I tell the man that I have this problem, then nine times out of ten, I probably won't get hired anyway. If I'm there at work and a tremendous thunderstorm comes up, then I've got to go, no matter what. I have just got to get out of there and get away; I can't function. As a matter of fact, I was working the other day and a thunderstorm came up and I almost fell off a ladder.

T. What were you doing?

C. I was hooking up an air line.

T. You were working for someone?

C. Yes.

T. Who were you working for?

C. Ajack Plumbing, Heating, and Electrical.

T. Do you have experience in this?

C. No. It's kind of a trade I'm in.

T. Is it an outside job?

C. Yes. I have my freedom. If a thunderstorm comes up, I can leave. He's the type of guy that would understand if I had to leave.

T. Does he know about your problem?

C. Yes.

T. Did you leave?

C. No. I was in a large building and it was just a quick one and it was only a few loud bursts and a few lightnings. It was one of those quick ones that comes over and goes away.

T. OK. Tell me what you did during this thunderstorm.

C. Well, I got down and started walking around.

T. You got down off the ladder?

C. Yes. I walked around looking for a cigarette and just sort of looking at the guy I worked with and grinned, and he knew what was wrong, so I just sort of walked around for a little bit. Like I say, it didn't stay there; it was just one of those quick ones.

T. What do you think when you are walking around?

C. Trying to calm myself down.

T. What are you telling yourself?

C. I tell myself, "Just be cool, don't let it get you."

T. What else are you saying when you get upset?

C. Well, I just think, "I wish to heck I wasn't like this." I'm trying to fight it and get it over with. I keep telling myself, "There is nothing wrong, what are you worried about?"

T. You're feeling anxious and you are angry with yourself because it's kind of annoying. What else are you saying?

C. It isn't like I am angry. It doesn't make me angry, but it makes me feel bad that I can't cope with it.

T. Now are you also saying, "I wonder when the next one is going to come?" And then when it does happen it frightens you? And then you calm down and you start waiting for the next one?

C. Well, I don't calm down. I guess I stay hyped up.

T. So are you saying also, "Gee, I wish this storm would get over," or "I wish it would go away?"

C. Yes. Actually, I'm thinking if I can only make it through *this* one.

T. What are you afraid you will do?

C. I'm afraid probably that my body reaction is going to overreact and I'm going to drop dead because my heart is pounding like everything.

T. So, you're telling yourself that, if I don't calm down, this anxiety is going to hurt me—kill me even.

C. Yes. I'm constantly trying to fight it when it does happen. I don't want to make a fool out of myself, like running out of a place, because I have done that before with my cousins and I don't want to appear that way to people.

T. What makes you think that this is going to be so severe that it will end in your dropping dead?*

C. Well, the feelings like the burning sensations, heart pumping, and so forth.

T. Do you think people can die from fright?

C. Yes. I think so.

T. Where did you learn that?

C. Well, I think the mind can conjure up anything, so to speak.

T. So, you're afraid that you will get so frightened and your body will respond so strongly that it will actually harm you and perhaps kill you?

*The fear that one can die from anxiety is common. Implosive clients need to be reassured that this is unlikely.

C. Yes. I believe it could happen.
T. Have you had anybody ever talk to you about that?
C. No. I like UFO's and psychology and became interested in it because of this. I don't know, I have always had the feeling that you can do just about anything that you want to do, if you try hard enough. I think if you get something in your head, it's hard to get it out.
T. So, you're afraid during these thunderstorms and during the time that you're really upset that you're hurting yourself and harming your body and that, if you don't get calmed down, there are going to be some permanent effects?
C. Well, I don't really know why I feel this way.
T. It's not so important what is true. What you say to yourself is important. We have to know what's going on at the time. . . Are you feeling that way at the time?
C. It's according to the severity of the storm or severity of what has happened. I can't pinpoint it. Like when it's a real thundering, deep-type storm, it's like I could just lay down. But if it's a mild storm, then I know that it is not quite as intense. I get the feeling that I could get away from it, if I had to.
T. What do you do if you are in a real bad storm? What are the techniques you use to reduce the anxiety?
C. Well, the only thing I can do is go to a place I know that is underground and I just go in there and order a drink and sit there and try to cope.
T. You go underground so you can't hear it?
C. Right. I guess that stems from jumping in a bunker. I don't know. It seems to be protective.
T. What are you thinking about when you are sitting there underground, drinking?
C. I'm just waiting for the storm to get over so I can calm back down.
T. Can you hear it while you are down there?
C. Yes. It's not as loud.
T. Do you feel safer?
C. A little. I guess so, that's where I go everytime or, at least, I try to get there. If I'm at home and I can't get somewhere or I am out in an open area, I just try to outrun it.
T. How do you outrun a thunderstorm?
C. I just look where the darkest clouds are or where the wind is blowing from and I'll go in the opposite direction. I watch where the flash is coming from and I'll try to go around it somehow.
T. You know intellectually that thunderstorms are not Vietnam mines and you know that there's little likelihood that you are going to be hurt, although there is some danger to the storms of lightning and thunder. Do you think about that?
C. No. I used to ride my bicycle in thunderstorms. I liked it.
T. You were hit by lightning once?
C. Yes.
T. So, the fact that you bring up thunderstorms and say, "This is when I'm really anxious," appears associated with some real fright based on past experience. Do you think of that?

C. Well, like I say, I get the same sensations from these three episodes. But I think the fear of the thunder and lightning is there now because I was with it I guess. But it is almost the same as when I was blown off the troop carrier. It was the same intensity.
T. Thunderstorms can be very frightening. In fact, you can be hurt in thunderstorms and loud sudden noises *are* frightening.
C. Well, the ones that really get to me are the ones with the deep, rumbling ones, low concussion-type thunderstorms where you see flashes of lightning jumping all over the place and the deep rumbling of the ground. Of course, they all bother me, but that really scares me the most.
T. OK. What's the name of the bars that you go to?
C. The Underground is one of them. I go to another one sometimes; it isn't underground but it doesn't have any windows at all. Usually there is someone to talk to.
T. Are they in the same town?
C. Yes. As a matter of fact, I moved close to the Underground for that reason.
T. Let's go back a little bit. What kind of things were problems for you when you were younger? What kind of things do you remember as being difficult?
C. Nothing, really. I really don't think I had any problems. I was athletic. I was outgoing and I could do just about anything I tried. I guess being poor was about it. Well, being poor never bothered me. I was just joking. I really can't think of anything that really bothered me.
T. Do you remember any early frightening experiences, such as early dreams, situations in which you were frightened? Sometimes children remember repetitive dreams, sometimes getting lost and not being able to find their way back to a safe place. Or any early experience at all that involved fright or fear.
C. I can't think of anything that really scared me.
T. Did you ever get hurt seriously when you were a child? Did you ever break any bones or have an accident?*
C. No. I fell on a spike when I was real little and it went in my throat, but I was only about 4- or 5-years old.
T. Can you tell me a little about that?
C. I was running in the yard and a long, thin railroad spike either went in my throat or my head. I can't remember which. Yes. It went in my throat.
T. Did it go through your mouth?
C. Yes. It stuck back in the roof of my mouth. But it didn't bother me that much. I just walked in and told my mother about it and pulled it out.
T. Do you remember anything else about that? It must have been unpleasant.
C. It is really amazing because I don't really remember being afraid or anything. It scared me, probably because I was young. I cried but, other than that, it didn't bother me.†

*Early pain experiences are often associated with later emotional experiences and should be incorporated into implosive scenes where appropriate.

†This is one of several statements that indicates that this client avoids and denies the significance of pain experiences.

T. You told me that your mother didn't punish you very severely. You said that once in a while she would use a hickory switch. You had no male authority over you. Your mother's boy friend was more like a friend and didn't exert much punishment, did not take the role of a father at all, as far as you're concerned.

C. I don't think so. I guess I looked to him as a man to respect, but I never really thought of him as my father. I pretty well had accepted what had happened with my father.

T. So, you don't recall ever being difficult or your mother having trouble with you particularly.

C. No.

T. Out of the three boys, were you the easiest to control, do you think?

C. No. I was probably the hardest.

T. Why?

C. I was rambunctious and hyperactive.

T. Did you ever take any medications for your hyperactivity?

C. No. I just use that as a term.

T. But you describe yourself as that way. Was that a diagnosis given by a doctor?

C. No. I was super-athletic. I got into everything. I played everything. I wanted to do everything. I wasn't afraid of anything.

T. Were you involved in all of the extracurricular activities in high school?

C. Not in high school. I had to work in high school.

T. You had to work?

C. Yes. I had to work in high school. I was small. I couldn't play that much anyway.

T. Did you have to support your mother then?

C. No. I just went to work. I was under the work-study program at school. I saw the chance to finish my high school plus work also and have some of the things that everybody else had. It's that simple, so I went to work.

T. How about early experiences with friends? Did you have a very good friend or two when you were younger?

C. Yes. I had a lot of friends.

T. Do you remember one or two guys that you really bummed around with a lot when you were younger?

C. When I was real young, there were John, Marty, and Ron. It was sort of like a group or a little club.

T. Do you still see them?

C. I haven't seen them in 15 years, at least.

T. Why don't you still see them?

C. I don't know where they are.

T. Did they leave the area?

C. John did. Ron is still around. I see him every now and then, but I really don't know where Marty is.

T. So these were buddies of yours before you went into the service?

C. Yes. This was when I was 12-or 13-years old.

T. How about when you were an older teenager?
C. Like I say, I knew everybody and everybody knew me. I won dance contests and things of this nature and everybody knew me.
T. Did you have someone that you trusted enough that you could sit down and tell anything to?
C. I think I had a couple of them. I have never been afraid to say anything. If I think it, I will say it.
T. Right now, is there someone you could sit down and tell everything to and feel comfortable?
C. Besides you, I don't think so . . . no.
T. You are seeing me professionally and that's a different thing. There is no one friend that you have had or have that you could sit down and talk with?
C. I've told a lot of people how I felt. Are you saying anybody that I could actually sit down with and tell anything to?
T. Anything that you've done in your past life.
C. I guess so. Several people.
T. But you don't have anyone that you do this with or that you talk to regularly in some intimate way?
C. Well, up until several weeks back, I talked with my girlfriend. I can usually talk to my mother, but I don't think I would if I had a real problem; I wouldn't because I wouldn't want to bother her with it.
T. Did you have any early repetitive dreams?
C. I have dreamed about things that have happened.
T. When you were young?
C. No. In the service. I dreamed once—I think I dreamed it, I'm not really sure—that I seem to remember my father bringing me something home and I was on the couch. I must have been about six or seven months old. It was a tractor or truck or something like that. Now, I don't know if I actually conjured that up or what or maybe it was my brother, but it seems like I remember that.
T. What's your earliest memory, other than that, that you are sure of?
C. The first thing that popped into my head was riding a bicycle around the house. I was about four or five. The second thing was driving my uncle's car when I was about 12. This is just what comes into my head, but it wasn't the earliest if I was 12. I remember the sixth grade at school.
T. So you don't have a lot of early memories that come into your mind right away when you say that?
C. No, I don't. As a matter of fact, I have a problem remembering people. A lot of people come up to me and I can't remember who they are until they tell me and give me some kind of background.
T. So you think you have a problem with memory?
C. Yes.
T. Remembering names?
C. Yes.
T. Have you always had that?

C. I don't remember. I don't mean to make a pun, but I really don't remember. I don't think I did. I was always very astute. Just the last couple of years I have sensed the fact that I just can't remember well anymore. As a matter of fact, when I was in Vietnam I forgot how old I was. I can understand being there and everything, but I actually forgot how old I was. I had to sit down and count it up. That was when I first started thinking about that. . .you know, that I don't remember things.

T. Perhaps we could test your memory to see. Have you ever had anybody do that?

C. No. I had reading comprehension tests and things like that, but I had no problem with them.

T. Nobody's ever given you a memory test?

C. Not that I know of.

T. So, you describe your early life as fairly full and interesting and you didn't have a lot of times when you felt down. You enjoyed it; it was normal in every sense. Did you have any problems as a juvenile with the law?

C. In the sixth grade me and all these guys formed a club. One of the guys had been around a little more than we had and we called the club the Vandals. We didn't even know what Vandals meant. We had the Police Chief come to school to talk to us. Ron did know what it meant. It was more of a joke than anything else because, when the Chief told us what it meant, we told him we would change it.

T. But you never had any time when you were arrested for anything?

C. No.

T. What is the worst trouble you have even been in?

C. DUI, I guess.

T. So you have had a ticket once for that?

C. Yes.

T. Do you drink everyday?

C. No.

T. When you do drink, do you tend to get drunk?

C. I have a low capacity. The time I got caught was because of my condition. It was late at night and nothing was open. The only place I knew that was open was 10–15 miles away. I went there and had a drink and was coming home and got caught. I really felt that I wasn't drunk, but the law said I was.

T. What problems do you have as a result of your injury in Vietnam? When you came here today, you mentioned that you were being photographed for a nose job to have some more plastic surgery done on your face. What other type of problems do you have besides that?

C. Well, I have had my knee operated on.

T. What was wrong with the knee?

C. It was all busted up. They took some parts out and put some more back in. I've got a lot of scars. I think the doctor said I have 52 scars on my legs, buttocks, and back. I have had two nose jobs. The machine gun smashed my nose. They did it once in the military and it didn't come out right. It hurt and there were a lot of problems. I couldn't breathe and I still can't. So they did it again here and the intern or whoever took the cast off snipped it here and here and here and pulled, and that disrupted everything because it made two holes in my nose, plus it messed up whatever they had done.

T. What are they going to do now?

C. I guess they are going to go back and patch up the holes and make it straight again.

T. What about the back problem?

C. I don't know what it is. I guess when I hit the ground several times, I hit hard.

T. Have you had any operations on your back?

C. No. I won't do that. They mentioned something about it, but I won't do it.

T. How does it interfere with your life?

C. Well, just sitting here now, it is starting to hurt. If I sit too long or if I walk too long or in a stable position too long, it hurts.

T. Does it get worse?

C. It bothers me every now and then. Just periods of time. Some mornings I find it hard to get out of bed. I sort of have to roll out and straighten myself up.

T. Is lifting a problem?

C. Yes. I lift from my arms mostly. I don't use my back, if I can help it.

T. But you don't avoid lifting?

C. No.

T. Now, I'd like to ask you some questions about your family. You've never been married?

C. No.

T. Have you ever thought about it?

C. Yes. I just don't believe I'm ready for it.

T. Why do you say that?

C. For one thing is this thing. As a matter of fact, I have had problems with my girlfriend because of this.

T. How is that?

C. This Underground place isn't exactly the best place to go. It's sort of a down-under type of place. She's fairly young and she just don't understand this like most people. I saw the problem arising, so I just told her it was just not right. I told her I had to do it, that I was sorry and could not help it.

T. So she objected to your going to the Underground?

C. Yes.

T. And you told her that was your safe spot?

C. I told her that she had to understand these things. I don't blame her. She just didn't understand.

T. How often do you go there?

C. Only when a thunderstorm hits. In the summertime, I'm there a lot.

T. So, it wasn't that you were going there to do anything else?

C. No. I wasn't going there to do anything. I was going there to hide.

T. And she objected to that?

C. Yes.

T. Why?

C. Well, like I said, it's not the nicest place in town.

T. But it doesn't seem to be that you were doing it that often. Would you leave her and go there?

C. Yes. I don't want her around there.
T. I'd think when you are feeling anxious, it would be nice to have someone close to you. What makes you feel this way?
C. I don't know. I just don't. I like to keep it to myself.
T. Most people, when they get very anxious, would find it comforting to have their girlfriend with them.
C. I don't know.
T. Wouldn't that be the average response? Most people, when they are anxious, like to have somebody around that they can trust. You're saying you're just the opposite of that.
C. Maybe I don't trust myself to be around somebody.
T. What do you think will happen?
T. Well, I almost had a wreck with a girl one time because of it and maybe that's the reason why. I told you about the time that I went up the side of the highway and she was in the car and it scared her. I realized that. She was about as nervous as I was by the time we got to the place we were going.
T. How many girlfriends do you think you have stopped seeing because of this problem?
C. I don't believe I have stopped seeing any of them for the problem, except the last one. I'm not saying that was the whole problem. There were other problems, but this contributed mostly to it, because of the fact that she just wasn't grown-up enough to understand and to accept.
T. Have you come close to having a relationship that could develop into marriage or living with a woman for a lengthy or extended period of time?
C. Yes. As a matter of fact, this last one was the only one I had ever gone with for a long time. I don't know. I enjoy my single life. That's all there is to it. But still, like any man, I want the things that marriage produces, such as kids. I just feel like people have to be ready and I just don't think I am.
T. What was the best part of your relationship with this woman? What did you like best about your relationship?
C. With this one?
T. Yes. Because you said that was one of the best relationships you have had.
C. Well, I had another that was just as good.
T. What was the best part of those relationships?
C. Well, every time I saw them, there was something new and, in the beginning, they were both super-understanding. I don't know. I just liked them. I liked their looks and the way they talked. I liked their domestic ideas, such as wanting to take care of the house and things of this nature. I don't know. I suppose it was their personality.
T. So you felt good when you were around them?
C. Yes.
T. And you wanted to be with them?
C. Right.
T. What were the things you could do, other than physical sex, that made you feel good?
C. I don't know exactly what you mean—Jenny was in Florida.

T. Jenny was the first one?
C. Yes.
T. What was the name of this last one?
C. Judy. I met Judy when I got out of service. She was the cutest little thing when I saw her. She was little and she seemed to be what I liked. She was too young and I knew it, so I let it go. Several years later, I met her again and we got to partying together and dating and it developed into something. I just enjoyed sitting at home watching T.V. Just everything from the beginning. I don't know if it got old or what. It got old when she started not understanding anymore.
T. Why did it interfere with your relationship so much?
C. In the beginning I only behaved strangely when there was a thunderstorm.
T. That wouldn't appear to be anything.
C. No. She noticed it right away. If an airplane would come over, I would jump off the couch. If a truck would start across the street, I would jump or a car door would slam. She could feel me every time something like that happened. If the television would flip, I would jump. So I told her what it was because I was waking up at night and she knew something was wrong.
T. Why were you waking up at night?
C. Dreams. I dream about it, also. In the beginning, it was all right. I could do as I pleased. We were just dating. After a while, I just kept giving up night after night. Before it was over, I gave up every night. I was going to school every night. I wasn't doing anything else, but actually playing marriage. That's all it was. After it got that far, then she started working on this problem . . . the fact that you "stay with me." She felt it was normal to want to be with somebody you love when you have this problem. But I don't. I don't know why. I just don't.
T. You said one reason was because you don't trust yourself when you're having this problem. Were you afraid you might hurt her?
C. I was not afraid I would hurt her but I was afraid that maybe indirectly something I did would hurt her. Like if I had a wreck or something.
T. Do you think there is any other reason why you want to be alone? You say you talk to the bartender?
C. Well, if somebody is in the back, I will talk to them. I will try to, anyway. Usually, I just go back and sit down by myself and sit there and do like this.
T. You have rhythmic movements?
C. Yes. Sort of like beating myself on my chest.
T. You beat yourself on your chest?
C. Yes. I know it doesn't do any good. I just do it. For some reason, it pacifies me. I get so up and I just do like this *(beats on chest)*. I sit there and laugh to myself. I try to humor myself.
T. Tell me about the dream that you have.
C. Well, it's just a recurring one of when I got blown up.
T. Do you ever see yourself dead?
C. No, not actually dead. Like I say, when I was blown-up, I felt that, so maybe I dream that but I don't actually dream I'm dead.

T. When do you wake up during the dream?

C. I have had dreams where my mouth just locked. I also have had dreams where I was dreaming that I was dreaming. I could wake myself up from the first stage but not the second one. In other words, the reality state.

T. Isn't that kind of frightening?

C. Yes. As a matter of fact, one night I was afraid to go back to sleep.

T. So the dream is really about being blown-up off the carrier?

C. Yes, most of the time.

T. Are there any other kind of dreams that bother you?

C. Well, I have a recurring dream. It's as if something is coming up like a black rubber line that is stretched out and I can knock it down with my feet or hands and it's not going to hurt me, but yet I just have to keep knocking it down or it will push me up. There is no fear there.

T. Anything else?

C. I think about bowling all the time. I think I think about it when I don't have anything else to think about; bowling pops into my head and I sit there and mentally bowl. I think what it is is that I bowled when I was little and I quit bowling and it seems like I'm trying to perfect it. It seems like I'm trying to get it exactly right.

T. So you are knocking some sort of line down and it reminds you of bowling?

C. Could be, I guess, It's coming up in between me. I know it won't hurt me or anything, but it just constantly comes. I can knock it down but it will still keep coming. It doesn't bother me or anything like that. Like I say, I think it takes the place of the fact that my mind is idle at the time and I don't have anything else to think about.

T. OK. I think I have a pretty good idea of where to start. I will be asking you questions as we go along. Now I would like to talk with you a little about what I propose we can do about this and ask you to do some exercises. First of all, frightening experiences like this can lead to having these kinds of responses, as you well know. This kind of reaction, we think, is due to kind of a basic conditioning. An anxiety reaction to specific things usually involves what we call "classical conditioning." That word is not important, but what it means is that, when you have similar experiences, you generalize to them and you respond in a very similar way as before. When your psychiatrist said to you, "It'll probably go away," he wasn't lying. Generally it does. The reason they go away, we think, is because people experience it over and over again and eventually it extinguishes or goes away. It's like, if you get thrown from a horse and you have a bad experience, you could be afraid of a horse, but the best way to deal with that, as everybody says, is to get back on the horse right away.

C. That's what gets me. That's the type of person I am. I wrecked my motorcycle when I was younger and it really hurt, but I just got back up and rode it. Anything I have ever done has been that way. But not this.

T. Animals are the same way. If a cat jumps on a hot, electric stove and burns its feet, the cat will stay away from that stove. The difference between the cat and a human is that the human can make the discrimination between a cold and hot stove. The cat will stay away from the cold stove, too. So the cat does not have the experience of the cold stove which would then serve to extinguish that response. We say he doesn't "test reality" unless you make him or put him there. Humans have this ability to think to such a degree that we can override the extinction. Sometimes it doesn't work. In this case, obviously, the usual extinction process has not worked. I have some ideas as to why that may be true, but I'm not certain. What I'd like to do is to have you imagine some experiences that perhaps you are avoiding that would help to "complete" this response and help to extinguish this response. I will also have you do some things in real life. Now these are not going to be altogether pleasant and it may even be that they will be very anxiety-provoking for you. But if you expose yourself to these situations enough times, we have good reason to believe that over a period of time you will come to feel relaxed in these situations that now make you anxious. Or if not relaxed, at least to the point where it isn't interfering with your life as it is now. One of the things I am concerned about is that you might be thinking, "This fear is going to drive me crazy eventually."

C. No. I don't think it will drive me crazy. I think it will hurt me when I get older. I don't think anything will drive me crazy.

T. Good. So, you don't have any feeling at all that, if you don't get over this, somehow it's going to have a real significant effect on your mind?

C. Well, maybe, I guess. I guess I have to think that, in a sense. Now I am begining to wonder anyway more and more. But I really don't think anything can drive me crazy, but I think if I had a bad enough experience, like if I got in one and couldn't get anywhere, maybe something would snap.

T. I assume that there is something that you're not presenting to yourself or something you're avoiding. Even though you're in situations with thunderstorms, there is something in your memory that is bringing this anxiety on. What I'd like to do is present these things to you and have you go through them in your imagination and see if we can bring that out. The other thing that humans do that animals don't do is that you can tell yourself that this is a scary situation and, if you tell yourself that, you can keep the anxiety going. One of the things that you're doing is telling yourself, "I'm afraid of thunderstorms" and it seems when you hear a thunderstorm or loud noise your reaction to it is anxiety-provoking, and what you say is, "Oh God, here it goes again" and when you say that, what you're doing is actually increasing that response. You're feeding into it. So you're making yourself anxious because you're anxious. Do you see what I'm saying?

C. Yes.

T. That's all well and good. I can talk about it and I can tell you how to understand what that is as soon as you start to feel the anxiety coming on. You start to get more anxious because you are afraid you're going to have this anxiety reaction. I can tell you that and you understand that but you say, "Well, I can't stop it; it still isn't going to help me."

C. I've tried.

T. So, we're going to try two methods. First we're going to flood you with these thoughts and experiences in imagination. I'm also going to ask you to do certain things when thunderstorms come up to try to get control of this. Second, we're going to talk about the way you think about these things and how they relate to your whole life. It seems to have gotten into very important things like your relationships with women, your job, and so forth.

Treatment

Therapy was carried out at three levels: (1) imaginal flooding for his fear of thunderstorms, (2) *in vivo* flooding for thunderstorms, and (3) implosive therapy aimed at the Vietnam experience including hypothesized fears of his own death. The following transcript is a portion of one of the scenes aimed at imaginal flooding.

T. You hear some things going on around you. You feel your weight pushing down into your chair. Concentrate on that. You can hear the sounds around you. It's very quiet.* Now I want you to imagine you are looking out my window. I want you to see the window. It's very high up. On the tenth floor. You can see for many miles. Just way off. Put your hand on the screens and feel the cool metal. Look out into the distance. You're seeing black clouds coming at you. It's a clear day but they are coming at you. You immediately respond as you see those clouds. There is a very very slight twitch in your chest. Your chest kind of tightens up. Feel that kind of warm sensation and you feel it just starting to swell up and your heart jumps a little bit. But you know you're in a safe place here even though it looks like it's going to storm. So just stand there and watch it. See the storm coming at you. It's coming closer. Black swirling clouds and you can see the lightning. Little sharp jolts of lightning but you can't quite hear it yet. It's getting closer as you stand there at the window. You feel like you want to run. But you can't. It's like you can't move. You're here and you have to stay here. I'm going to let you stay here in the office. See that? See the storm coming closer and closer? Pay attention to your bodily sensations. Just watch that and fantasize. Feel those tensions. That's right. Feel that tension in your chest. Feel the storm coming up now. You can even hear it. It starts to blow against the windows now and they rattle. Then you hear a first clap of thunder. Hear it starting again. A low rumbling sound. Getting closer. Finally, a real loud clap and you can see the lightning come across the sky; it seems almost to touch the building because we are up so high. And you can't get out. You go to the door and you

*This first scene is a good example of how implosive therapists use fears that bodily sensations can be harmful, and may even be critical.

grab it. Feel the doorknob. You start to pull. You want to get out of here but you can't. Just stay here and face it. You stand here and feel the thunderstorm coming all around you and the clouds clap louder and louder and it crashes around you. It reminds you of your time in Vietnam and you think about that now. When you were on the troop carrier and you start to think about that as you watch this thunderstorm. You feel that sensation. Hear it. Feel it. You're in the middle of it. You start to get very anxious. Tighter and tighter in your chest. Your heart is pounding now. Getting more and more anxious. You feel the back of your head stiffen up. Concentrate on those bodily sensations now. See the storm around you. It engulfs you. You are standing here looking out and finally you hear a loud crack. Then the lights go off and you can feel that. You feel it blowing through the window and the window opens up. Feel it. It blows you back against the wall. You feel the cold rain and wind. It starts to blow the books around the office. Upsets the desk now and you flatten out against the wall. Feel the terror in that. Finally, you feel the pressure of the wind against your chest. Blowing on your chest very hard. Pushing you and pushing you up against the wall. Holding you there. You can't move. It's so powerful. Like a vacuum. Feel yourself being blown so hard against the wall that the wallboard actually starts to crack and you fall down on your back and you can't move. The pressure of the wind is so great and the thunder and the lightning all around you is great. Finally, you find yourself getting dizzy and you start to get dizzier. You start to feel the darkness coming over you. It's getting darker. You feel yourself passing out. Darker and darker and you can't think. You can't even think who you are. You just have this swirling and whirling feeling all around you and you're just going completely out. It's now like you are in a long tunnel and you hear the sounds around you and you feel the pressure but you can't move. You don't have any control over your body. You can't make your muscles move. You are aware of things and you can hear things but you can't see. There is a blackness. You can smell. The smell of something burning. Everything is totally dark. You can't talk. You can't move. You can only hear something. Think about the bodily sensations you have as you go deeper and deeper into it. Feel the black, cold rain. Hot chest flashes. Your heart starts to pound faster and faster. Finally, you start to feel a stab. A painful stab in your chest, in the left side of your chest. You push back against the ground. Then things go completely blank. You just kind of ease the grip. You can't hold any longer. It's as if you are dying. You are so frightened, scared, anxious, and so upset that you start to pass out. Feel that pain in your chest. It's just too much. Your body just crumples and you're dying. Feel yourself. Feel that slipping, slipping, slipping away feeling. Losing control. Losing all control and you are dying. Feel it. The pain in your chest. You can't breathe well. You start to gulp for air and there isn't any. Feel heat all around the crashing sounds. You start to swirl around through the tunnel deeper and deeper. You start to feel very scared. You're dying. The only thing that you can start to experience now is that CRASH, CRASH, CRASH. Feel it. Pay

> attention to those bodily sensations now. Concentrate on them. Concentrate on your heart pounding. Let it pound away. Pound away. Concentrate on those warm feelings as you just slip away. Then some attendants come along and they just pick up that limp body and you can hear them and they're going to put you into a cart and carry you off. Hear the hearse coming. Kind of rumbling along. You're aware of all this but you can't speak. They can't hear you. Evidently, they think you're dead. They just kind of carry you off, put you in a casket, and they put you in the ground. You feel yourself getting lowered into that cold ground. You hear the squeak and squeak of the pulleys as they lower you down in that box. Everything's kind of dark. You haven't got any control. Here the dirt comes. Coming on top of you in the casket. They are burying you. You feel the pressure of the dirt pushing down on the casket. You can't breathe very well. You're just buried right there. You can't move. No control. Concentrate on that lack of control. Complete helplessness. Not being able to move. You can't move your arms or your legs. You can't even think very straight. You can't carry out a thought. You're totally helpless. Helpless. Get into that. Feel it. Concentrate on those bodily sensations. Feel that storm. Hear it all around you. You can't move. You're totally out of control. No bodily functions. Nothing working.

At the second treatment session we used the following implosive scene. This is an excerpt from a memory scene, and therefore involves more client input. This scene taps his war experience, but notice the similarities between this and the former scene with regard to suggested bodily sensations.

T. You're going on a mission. I want you to imagine that you are there. Try to get into it now. Imagine it as clearly as possible. Come on and get into it now. It will be as if you are really there. We will try to continue with it and I will have you do some things that are different than what really happened, but I want you to work along with me. So go ahead and tell me what's happening. I want you to imagine it as you tell it. You can even use the present tense. Such as, "We are on the road and I am on . . ."

C. Well, we were supposed to be on standby but we took a couple of days off. We got permission and we had to leave early that morning—about 6:00 A.M. We went down the same road.

T. Can you see the road now?

C. Yes, plain as day.

T. You can feel the thump, thump along as you are riding. Where are your hands?

C. On my machine gun.

T. Is it a warm day?

C. Hot. Heat's coming up from the motor, too.

T. Bouncing along you see your friends around you. How do you feel right now?

C. Tense. Seems like you always know when something's going to happen.* We were talking and everything until we got out of the AO, but now we were all quiet. Like the feeling that we all knew something was wrong. We are just riding along.

T. Feel that now. The warm tension mounting. Anxiety. Feeling of concern. You're on guard. You start up the road and what happens then. You're going down the wrong road, aren't you?

C. Yes. We passed the V-shaped road. I just shrugged my shoulder like, "I don't know." He calls up front and asks, "Are we going the wrong way?" We were going the wrong way and he knew it. So he reversed march. We sat there for about 2–3 minutes.

T. Did he get a kick out of that?

C. Huh?

T. Does he get a kick out of that? Did he pick that up and tell the chief?

C. I don't know. Well, he was kind of an uppity guy anyway. He had been there a long time and he was sort of the head of the group. Well, not the head but sort of an overbearing type guy and he probably got a kick out of telling him we were right and he was wrong. The sargeant we had at that time wasn't too up on what was going on because he had just got over there and everything.

T. Can you see yourself sitting there and waiting for the order to come to reverse? How does it come down?

C. Well, after we had done that I think we came back and we reversed march and we looked at each other kind of funny because it would have been just as simple to go around the block. It didn't really matter that much. This is actually the first time we had ever done that. First and last, by the way. We backed up into some tall weeds and bushes and turned around and headed back down the road and took a left down the original road we were supposed to go down.

T. Can you see yourself turning now ahead of the column?

C. Yes. We all turned around and then lined back up again with us in front. We had the feeling that something was going to happen. I sat up out of my hole a little further than usual. The guys on top could tell they were getting ready for something. There was just a feeling in the air. You get to where you just know. But we didn't know it was going to be what it was. We thought it was going to be an ambulance or something. We started back down into the road we were supposed to and just as we were going under a tree—BOOM!

T. OK. I want you to feel this now. You can feel this in slow motion. You can hear that tremendous crash. It just keeps reverberating. Everything slows down now.† You see a flash getting bigger and bigger. The noise sounds like

*Notice how the client lapses into the present tense. This should be encouraged.

†The "slow motion" suggestion sometimes helps to magnify the imaginal experience.

thunder and it rumbles louder and louder. The pressure is pushing against you and you feel yourself losing control. Losing control and you are out of control and things start to go black. Your eyes are dim and you can't hear anything and you feel yourself floating. Floating and sailing into the air. You must be dying. You are dying. Feel that. Float into air. Feel that floating sensation. You can hear all your buddies yelling and screaming and see all of them. I want you to see the way it was. You can see them there now all bloodied and you can feel your hot face and chest. You know that you had been hit too and you don't even know if your body is in one piece. It's as if it is flying apart. You are flying apart. Out of control. Concentrate on that. You're losing your grip. Floating and feeling the floating sensation. You are dying. "I am dying, I'm dying. . . ." You look down where you are and you are ripped apart.* You don't have any arms, you don't have any legs and you can see the bloody stumps. You are just totally ripped apart and your stomach is ripped apart. You feel your eyes, nose, and mouth bleed. You're just destroyed. You are destroyed and you are dying. You are gasping for air and you can't see. All you can feel is the numbness now. You are blacking out and you can look down now as you float and see this massacre and see all of the dead bodies until you just THUD . . . hit the ground. It is the last thing you feel before you just pass out. You're dead. You're dead. What do you feel? The pain starts all over again. The pain is coming back. That's what you feel as you lay there dead. Hot, hot burning pain. It starts again, that floating feeling. You see your body again. Torn apart. Totally destroyed. Blown apart. No legs or arms and you float. You see them all kind of floating around you there. All the dismembered parts of your body just floating around you. You feel that THUD again. Then they lay there. Ugly. Feel yourself. Losing control beyond your legs. They aren't attached anymore. Then you die. Again, it seems like you feel the pain coming back again. It just goes on and on. See all the bloody bodies around you. You are in a pool of your buddies' blood. All of them dying, dead, screaming, "Help me, help me." You can't move. You can't do anything. You don't do anything. They are looking at you like they're begging for help. You feel it. You've got to do something. Somehow you feel like you caused all this.† You were really responsible. You could've done something about it. Do you feel that responsibility? They all look at you and you just deny it. "No, no I'm not responsible." But you feel it. Sometimes it feels that way. Sometimes you wonder if you could have done something about it. Somehow you might have been able to stop all that. You feel that responsibility and the guilt. You see the pools of blood around you. Black,

*The therapy goes beyond reality to clients' fears.

†If guilt is associated with the memory, this should help bring it out. The therapist must wait for the client's response and question him later.

brown, and white skin is all around you. It makes you sick to your stomach. You feel very bad. Just go through that again. Now let's really feel that feeling. You're there and you're going down that road. You can feel that thump along and you've got your hands on the cold steel. It's very hot. You move on down the road and finally you see that you are passing up that fork. See that fork. You've missed it. You know it. Call up. "Aren't we going the wrong way?" Order comes to halt. Wait. You start to feel something's up. You reverse. You turn around and start down the road. Feel the heat and you start to get anxious. You know that something's up. You get up and you watch. You're very tight and tense. You sit up higher and you turn the corner back and you know that it's coming. You feel something but you don't know what. Then, THUD, BLAST! A fiery blast. The pressure. The heat. The blinding, blinding heat and light. It deafens you. Everything pushes back on you and you start to float and you start to fly. You're flying slowly and the pressure and the heat in the chest build up. You feel that now. You are there again. You feel your body coming apart and you look around you and your body seems to be dismembered as if you have no legs or arms. You can't see, you can't hear. You see all of this below you now. All of your buddies around you. They look up at you as if to say you knew something. Feel that responsibility. Feel and see yourself torn apart and bleeding. Blind and deaf. Your legs and arms are now floating around you. And finally, THUD, HIT. A pool of blood around you tells you everything is a mess. Totally destroyed. Broken limbs, bushes, pieces of tanks and B-100's all over the place. Just totally destroyed. You are feeling bad. You're dying. You must be dead. You can't move. You feel it now. Feel all that. Pay attention to any bodily sensations you have now and hold onto them, in the chest area, especially, as long as you can until they're gone. . .

In vivo flooding took the form of homework. When a thunderstorm was about to begin, George was instructed to go outside and imagine that he was being hit by lightning and at the same time review the experiences he had in Vietnam. He was told to experience the anxiety and not to retreat from it until he felt comfortable.

The imaginal scenes were repeated three times each in the therapist's office and he was instructed to practice them at home. After two months of *in vivo* practice in which six thunderstorms occurred, George did feel that he had gained control over his anxiety. He stated that he still did not like thunderstorms but "could stand them." A year later he was still working full-time on an outside job, and was able to stay on the job during the threat of thunderstorms, although he continued to feel some anxiety during storms. George used *in vivo* flooding as a means of controlling his anxiety. By the time of his last follow-up session, he was going to school part-time taking drama classes.

Case Study

Posttraumatic stress disorder is not specific to a war experience. In fact, most neurotic problems tend to result from past stress (i.e., aversive-conditioning experiences). The next case example involves traumatic experiences during boot camp rather than a war experience.

Bryan, a 29-year-old separated male, was admitted to the hospital complaining of multiple symptoms of anxiety and anger. These symptoms began 11 years ago when Bryan was in the marines at boot camp for only 29 days. During that time, his drill sergeant was reported to have traumatized him in several ways. The sergeant would yell in his face and criticize him and his family, causing him great fear. The sergeant reportedly locked Bryan in a small stand-up locker and left him there alone for hours, kicked Bryan in the chest, and kicked Bryan's legs out from under him. Since the boot camp experience, Bryan said he had suffered much anxiety, had regularly thrown-up blood, had nightmares of being locked in the locker, was claustrophobic in any closed-in spaces, and suffered severe headaches. In addition, anytime the back of his head was hit, he would "black out" and violently fight with people around him. He, in fact, had a history of many fights. He also had been unable to hold a job for more than one or two months, generally leaving after feeling dominated by, and fighting with, his supervisors. His anxiety was further exacerbated when his wife unexpectedly left him a few months prior to admission.

Bryan was the youngest of three children and he described a normal, active, outgoing childhood. Of possible significance was the fact that his father was an alcoholic who became violent and abused his mother. Bryan's parents divorced after he left home.

In designing a treatment for Bryan, we accepted his assessment that his traumatic experiences in boot camp were the root of his symptoms. Implosive scenes began in the third therapy session and basically replayed the aversive experiences, with the additions of the expression of rage towards the sergeant, experiencing the feared loss-of-anger control, as well as body mutilation, being trapped, death and rejection/desertion. The first several sessions focused primarily on fear of the sergeant and of the stand-up locker. Later sessions focused more on the expression of anger and on fears of desertion.

Reproduced below is the fifth session. Note that two therapists are present. In teaching the technique, we often do cotherapy, with the student gradually taking a more active role. The session begins with a discussion of the homework scene and continues with a scene presentation in the office. Note that the scene begins as a replay of traumatic events that had actually happened, with the therapist playing the role of the abusive sergeant, and even poking Bryan lightly to recreate the sensations of the sergeant poking him.

T1. How are you doing?
C. OK. I just woke up. I have been having a busting headache but now it's starting to ease off some.
T1. Are you going to be able to do this?
C. I'm going to try.
T1. Tell me about your homework. How did it go?
C. OK., up until we got around to being buried in the hole, then it didn't go too good.
T1. Were you able before that to imagine the sergeant dressing you down?
C. Yeah.
T1. Could you imagine yourself getting angry back?
C. Yeah.
T1. Were you able to verbally tell him off?
C. Yeah.
T1. Were you able to punch him?
C. Uh, yeah, but not that much. To me, it is still hard to do it.
T1. How about when he then attacked you?
C. Yeah, that was fairly easy because, you know, he actually attacked me before. But when we got down to imagining him beating me to death and my being buried in the ground, I kept losing it then.
T1. Could you see him beating you to death?
C. Oh, yeah. He kept beating on me but, when it got down to being put in the hole and all that, I couldn't keep it.
T2. You mentioned the last time about being in the coffin. Could you see yourself in that?
C. Uh, yeah, a little bit. I mean, it wasn't, I would say, as clear as the other. As soon as I started with him beating back on me and everything like that, I started getting a little nervous. Started losing the image a little bit.
T1. Did you keep track of when you did your homework and what your ratings were?
C. I wrote it all down. I did one Monday right after I left here. Like I say, it worked out pretty good, up until the point where I got towards the end.
T1. How much anxiety or emotion would you say you had on it?
C. Oh, considerable, especially getting down to the point with having to think of him beating me, you know, that bad.
T1. Where would you put it on our 0–100 scale?
C. Oh, close to 100 as far as being nervous.
T1. So you did one on Monday and did some Tuesday?
C. Yes, I did one on Tuesday afternoon and then one late Tuesday evening.
T1. Where would you rate those in terms of emotion?

C. Both at about 95.
T1. And this is Wednesday, have you had a chance to do a scene today?
C. No, because like I said, I've had a headache.
T1. OK. Well, let's go ahead and try the scene again. Just close your eyes and picture the sergeant down there at the end of the line.
C. Yeah, in the barracks, he's walked in.
T1. And he comes right to you this time. He doesn't mess around. He comes right up to you. What does he say?
C. He starts jumping all over me, you know, hollering and screaming.
T1. That's right. He's hollering and screaming all the time. "You puke, you son of a bitch," and then he starts talking about your family. His breath is right there and you can start to feel the tension build-up. Right there, he is on you. Why does he do all this to you? Why does he do all this to you? He keeps calling you a puke and a son of a bitch, and he would just as soon kill you as to look at you. "Your mother is a lousy lay." Some of the other recruits that he does it to, you can see that they are kinda clutzy, aren't they?
C. Some of them, some them aren't.
T1. I wonder why he picks on you and that thought goes through your mind too a lot, doesn't it?
C. Yeah.
T1. Why is he always picking on you? For some reason, he hates you, doesn't he? He hates your guts and he's telling you that right now—"you son of a bitch, you puke," and he just keeps calling you names. Standing right there—he's right on you. "You bastard! You puke! Your mother is a lousy lay," and then he starts poking you in the chest. "You shit bag! You puke! Shape up, private! God damn it! I'll send you to Motivation, you uncoordinated son of a bitch. I'm going to screw your mother and your sister, even though they are lousy lays. You're from a long line of bastards. Your father was a bastard. You are a bastard. Your sister sells it on the street. Doesn't she, private?"
C. No sir.
T1. "Yes, she does. I'm going to make a marine out of you, private, or I'm going to kill you. You god damn puke." And he just keeps on talking like that. On and on and on, and then he pokes you again and says, "you puke, you son of a bitch." His face is right there. "You puke! You son of a bitch! Your mother, your father," and on and on and on. "I would like to kill you. I would kill you in a heartbeat. Your mother is a lousy lay. Your father is a bastard. Your sister sells it. She is a lousy lay, too. And you are a bastard, too. You son of a bitch. You puke! You are a puke private, aren't you?"
C. No, sir.
T1. "You are a puke private," and he moves on and then you call him a name. Go ahead, call him a name.*

*Up to this point, the scene has been basically a replay of actual past events. Here, we begin to elicit the feared anger response toward the sergeant, something that never occurred in boot camp, but has been occurring in misplaced form ever since.

C. Son of a bitch.
T1. Say it again.
C. You son of a bitch.
T1. Then he comes back over and says, "What did you say, private?" And you say, "I said you are a son of a bitch, sergeant."
C. You are a son of a bitch, sergeant.
T1. And he says, "What did you say, private?"
C. I said you are a son of a bitch, sergeant.
T1. And you see his face right there. Do you see his face? Let's re-run that. He's just gone off of you and the words come right out of your mouth. See him down there and you hate his guts and you say, "You son of a bitch!"
C. You son of a bitch!
T1. And he comes back and he says, "What was that? You puke, what was that?"
C. You son of a bitch.
T1. You are the son of a bitch, private.
C. You are a son of a bitch.
T1. You are, private.
C. You are.
T1. You are a puke.
C. No, sir.
T1. Yes, you are. I am going to send you to Detention or Motivation for talking back to me. You know that, don't you, private?
C. Yes, sir.
T1. Is that what you want, private?
C. No, sir.
T1. Would you like to say you are sorry, private? You say, "No, sir, you puke". Tell him that.
C. No, you are a puke.
T1. Do what you want with me 'cause you're a puke. Tell him that.
C. Do what you want 'cause you're a puke.
T1. Do you see his face when you're saying that to him? What does he look like?
C. Angry.
T1. That's right. He's really angry. You have really got him mad. He pulls you out of line now. He pulls you out of line and he doesn't mess with the locker this time. The locker is too good for you. That's just punishment. He is going to kill you, that's right, he's going to kill you right now. He tells you that and he looks at you and he says, "You are dead, puke. I told you I would kill you in a heartbeat and this is it." And then he takes you and he smacks you real hard in the chest and he shoves you down. Kicks you in the neck, kicks you in the stomach. You can feel the harm done inside your body—the organs bursting. And then he stands you up and he slams you against the wall. Feel that? You see him slamming you against the wall and then you strike back and you say, "You god damn son of a bitch. I'll kill you first."

C. You god damn son of a bitch. I'll kill you first.

T1. That's right and then you say it again, the same thing again. A little louder this time.

C. You god damn son of a bitch! I'll kill you first!

T1. And then you take your fist and you smack him. See his face in your mind's eye and then you smack him. Move your fist in the air. Good. And then you slam him against the lockers. Take him, he's going to kill you, take him with both your hands and you slam him against the lockers. That's right. Slam him again. And then he hits you and kicks you in the groin and he kicks you in the stomach and he's all over you. He's a quick, strong, son of a bitch, isn't he? And he hates your guts. And you get the feeling that he is better than you. He's stronger than you. He's quicker than you and he's meaner than you and he's just all over you now. He's smashing your face. Your teeth are falling out. Your tongue is half bit off. Your belly is distended from the busted organs in there. Your groin is aching and he's smashing your legs. Tearing your face—your skin is hanging off of you. You're a mess! And all the time he is calling you names—son of a bitch, bastard, and I'll screw your mother after you are gone; I'll screw on your grave. And he just keeps on hitting you and calling you names. And then he pulls you up again and throws you against the wall and you strike back again. "You god damn bastard, I don't care what happens to me, I'm going to kill you. I don't care. I'm going to kill you," and you hit him again. Hit him again! Hit him again and again and again. *(Bryan punches in the air.)* That's right. You just keep hitting him again and again. Do you see him there? He's right there in front of you. That's good. And then he tears you limb from limb and it's a big brawl. You're hitting him and he's kicking you, you're kicking him and now he's down on the ground and you stomp him with your foot. "You son of a bitch." Stomp him. *(Bryan stomps ground.)* That's right. Stomp him again. Stomp him again. And then he picks you up again and throws you against the locker and he smashes your head against the locker. You fall on the floor and he's on top of you now. He's smashing your head, smashing your head, smashing your head and then you get up somehow and something snaps in your mind that you have got superhuman strength. You pick that big sergeant up and you throw him on the floor. You see that? Throw him on the floor and then you walk over and kick him in the head. He's got this grin on his face, this grin on his face. You walk over and you kick him in the head. You stomp that grin. You see that? Stomp that grin. That's right. Again. Again. Again. *(Bryan stomps floor.)* "I hate you, you son of a bitch. You're the son of a bitch."

C. I hate you, you son of a bitch. You're the son of a bitch.

T1. That's right. Stomp him again and again and again. All of a sudden, you stomp him one last time and the blood is coming out of his mouth and he makes a weird sound and he dies. He dies. You've killed him. You're bleeding but he's dead. He's dead and then they come and they lock you up. They lock you up. You don't go to Motivation. You don't go to Casuality Company.

They lock you up and you are behind bars. See that? The bars and the walls around you—it's not a very big cell, is it? There's a potty in there, a bunk—it's tight. You can't get out. You hear those bars close and you're trapped. You're really trapped and you've killed him. You killed him and it's your fault. He was just trying to do his job. He was trying to make a marine out of you but you killed him. Stomped him to death. Lost control. Mouthed back and then you killed him and the bars are there and the walls are there and everything. And then the next thing you know, you are in the court and they are telling about what you did to this man. They're showing pictures of him—his body all mutilated—and then the judge sentences you and he says, "death." And they take you away and they put you in a small cell again and you are stuck there waiting to be executed. Can you picture yourself there in that cell? A murderer—no chance of getting out. No one comes to see you. You don't know if they don't care or if they can't get in or if they don't know, but no one comes to see you. They shove some food once in a while through the slot. No one will talk to you because they hate you. What kind of thoughts go through your mind?

C. Fear.

T1. What kind of thoughts go through your mind?

C. Fear and being nervous.

T1. You have done it now, haven't you? You have gone and done it. You're in a small cell and the only place you are going to get out to is a small coffin. How are they going to kill you? How are they going to execute you?

C. Gas chamber.

T1. Gas chamber and you're strapped down in that chair right now and you can't move. You're trapped in that chair and the gas comes in and you can't get your breath and your muscles are tight. Your heart is pounding and you can just see that sergeant's face smiling now 'cause he's got you planted. You're trapped and you're dying and the next thing you know you are in that box—the lid is open but you're in that box. You feel those sides around you and you have some kind of a quicky burial ceremony which nobody comes to, and then they slam the top shut and it's dark, and then you hear the creak as they lower your coffin down into the dark, cold ground—inch by inch and lower and lower—the tight box around you—darkness around you, feel it, down lower and lower, creak, creak, creak and then thud—the bottom of the hole and the dirt starts coming in and you hear that—each shovelful thumping on top of the coffin—6 feet under, 6 feet of heavy dirt, inside of a box, tightness, coldness, dampness, loneliness, no one cares and you are trapped there, trapped there never to get out, never to get out. Totally trapped and no hope. No place to run. No one to strike. Just that box and you and the dirt above you. You feel a cold, damp chill come over you and you realize that you will never get out. You are trapped—it's tight around you. Do you feel that sensation? What kind of thoughts go through your mind?

C. Fear, just fear.

T1. Where do you notice the fear?
C. All over.
T1. Do you notice it in your stomach? How about your arms?
C. My stomach is flip-flopping.
T1. Stomach flip-flopping. What else?
C. Feel a little shaky, edgy.
T2. Feel cold?
C. Yes.
T2. Kind of chilling, isn't it? Down your back. There is no way out. I mean, even if you could open the coffin, there are still 6 feet of dirt.
T1. What are you going to do?
T2. Nothing, this is it. You're trapped. It's over. It's over. Right now. The end.
T1. And it goes on and on. All your options are over and you are trapped. Trapped and the fear ripples through you—there is nothing you can do. You can't move. You can't move even a little bit. You're dead and you can't move. You're trapped. There is no way out—those four walls tighter and tighter around your passive body, darkness and not a smidgen of light and no one will ever touch you again. You will never feel water on your lips and tongue again, never eat again, never have warmth. Cold. Thirsty. Hungry. Alone. No one cares, and hours pass, days, weeks. Weeds are growing on your lawn and no one cares; months, years, decades, hundreds of years, two hundred years, three hundred years, four hundred years—you've been in that tight box—tight around you for four hundred years—cold, shaking for four hundred years, aware of the cold and the aloneness. Absolutely no pleasure. No caring. No one cares about you. You lost control. You hurt somebody. You killed somebody. Feel that tight box. Tight. Tight. It's dark. What kind of thoughts go through your mind? Years have passed and you just lay there, trapped in your own body inside of the coffin under the ground. Feel that lid right up above you as close as the sergeant was to you. That lid is there.
T2. The darkness never ends—always dark.
T1. And you're dead and you're under the ground.
T2. It's a cramped feeling worse than that locker was.
T1. Feel it?
C. I'm starting to lose it.*
T1. Well, let's back it up. You're sitting in the gas chamber—you're in the chair. Feel that? You have killed the sergeant and you're in the gas chamber. You just look around at some bare room—you see nothing—just a bare room and you feel yourself sitting in that chair. Feel the chair on your bottom against your back there and then you hear the gas—ssssss—just keeps coming and you can feel your body starting to spasm as it dies. And it's like you can see yourself sitting there and being there at the same time,

*Loss of image clarity here is hypothesized to result from fear. Therefore, the scene content is thought relevant and the therapist repeats it.

and the gas comes in and it slowly, slowly kills you and you are trapped in that chamber and then they unstrap you from the chair and you're dead. And they take you and you feel a little better almost because they are carrying you and touching you, and then they put you into this cold box. They throw you into this box and you feel yourself dumped in that box. Do you see that? See it. You're really dead and you're really in that box. You don't want to be there but you are, and there is nothing you can do about it. You're right there and it's all around you, it's all around you and you feel like you can't get your breath, your muscles are tight and the box is around you, tight, tight, tight. And the lid comes down. Smash! Right in your face. The darkness hits you and the coldness comes on. The coldness, the loneliness and the box all around you and you are trapped tighter than ever before. There is no way to get out. You are really trapped this time. There is nothing you can do and it's going to go on and on and on and then they lower you down into the hole. You hear those last noises—the creak of the pulleys as they lower you down—the dirt comes on, shovelful by shovelful and then there is nothing, nothing. You're alone in that box and it's cold. You can feel the sides and you can see darkness, darkness because the box is all around you. There is nothing to see, but you can feel that box and fear throughout all your body, your stomach and your muscles, your head, your chest, breathing all fearful and it just goes on and on and on and on. You feel that box around you now. Don't block it out. Feel that box. You are all alone and you are dead. Can you see yourself dead inside that box?

C. Not clearly, no.*

T1. OK., see it unclearly. Just feel it around you. Years pass, hundreds of years, hundreds of years, all alone and no one cares. No one cares. They never dig you up. You never get out of that box. You are trapped. Trapped. Trapped. Dead in the coffin in the ground. Cold ground. The coffin doesn't rot—it's a good coffin and there is no way out. Just always in that box. You wished they had cremated you but you are in that box. Feel it on your feet—the bottom of the box—the box on your head. What part of that can you picture?

C. I can't get any of it that clear.

T2. What feelings do you have right now?

C. Very nervous and sick to my stomach.

T1. Being stuck in that box—it's hard to picture because there is nothing to see—it's just black. But you know you're in that box. You can know that you are in that box. Stuffiness. Coldness. Tightness. You know that you are in that box because you feel the anxiety of being in that box. There is no way out. It goes on and on and on. You wish it would end but it doesn't. It goes on and on and on—hundreds and thousands of years—dead for eternity. Eternity—

*Even though the client continues to have difficulty imaging the scene, he appears to be quite anxious and the therapist continues, confident that with repetition image clarity will improve.

that box will last forever. You are trapped. Never get out—never, never. Two thousand years, 24 hundred years, 3,000 years, the box is with you, around you, tight. Box—you're in the box. It's locked—you are trapped. There is no way out. Four thousand years. Tight, darkness. There is only you in that box. You in that box alone. Tightness, cramped. You in that box. No way out. Feel it all around you.

C. I think I am getting it.

T1. OK., you can open your eyes. I think you are getting it. You wouldn't be anxious if you weren't in the box.

T2. You are having a reaction.

C. My headache is coming back now.

T2. You know what they say, no pain, no gain.

C. Yeah. *(Laughs)*

T2. You know, I had a couple of observations today. This was the first time that I've seen that you were able to get into hitting the sergeant. You've kind of come over that milestone today. Are you feeling that?

C. Yeah, but not as much as I think I should. It's a little easier to swing but as far as, you know, actually picturing it, it's not as clear to me as I think it should be.

T2. Is the clarity improving?

C. Yeah, today was pretty good.

T2. With the swinging, I'm talking about.

C. Yeah, a little better than in the past. It's getting a little better every time.

T1. Where would you rate the clarity of the first part of the scene where he is calling you names?

C. Oh, I can rate that real high.

T1. How high?

C. 70 or 75.

T1. How about the part where you call him names?

C. A little less, because I still have a little bit of a block against that.

T1. How about the part where you are fighting him?

C. That's a little less, too. About 50, maybe a little bit more. It's better than what it was.

T1. How about where you are in jail?

C. No, as soon as you start talking about those closed-in spaces and everything, it seems like I have trouble picturing it. I would rate it less than 50.

T1. What would it be just for comparison purposes?

C. 40.

T1. And how about when you are in the gas chamber?

C. Same thing, 40.

T1. How about in the coffin?

C. That was even less, about 20.

T1. Even though you can't see it too well, can you feel it?

C. Yeah, I must see it because I get very nervous. Yeah, I can feel it. I can feel it so I must be getting into it.

T1. Well, the visualization is only one part of it, and there are all the other senses so you feel them in other ways.

C. I must be.
T1. You looked like you were feeling something.
C. Sweat coming on me then.
T1. Muscles tight.
C. Yeah, I think I broke my little finger. *(Laughs)*
T1. We don't want that.
C. Yeah, I can feel that. I just can't see it too well.
T1. Well, that's the important thing, the image will come gradually.
C. As soon as you started talking about it, I started breaking out in sweat.
T1. OK., again use the whole basis of therapy as homework. Get as many practice sessions as you possibly can. We'll see you next week.

Bryan was discharged from the hospital after 7 implosive therapy sessions, and was followed for 7 additional sessions as an outpatient. In addition, since his headaches did not respond to implosive treatment, he attended 5 sessions of a stress management group that resulted in a substantial decrease in headache frequency. His other symptoms largely resolved and these gains were maintained at a 6-month follow-up. He reported feeling calmer; had had no nightmares, blackouts, or fights; was able to function when necessary in tight spaces; and had been employed since a few weeks after discharge. At one point, he had an increased level of anxiety and irritability when he had to appear in court for a minor violation and feared that he might be imprisoned. This anxiety, however, was temporary and did not result in nightmares or fights.

Simple (Specific) Phobia

Simple phobia is defined as a persistent, irrational fear that results in a desire to avoid a specific object or situation. It is distinguished from agoraphobia and social phobia as the latter are more general fears of places and people (defined later in this chapter). Simple phobias, sometimes referred to as specific phobias, are relatively common. They usually involve fears of animals, particularly dogs, mice, snakes, or spiders. Most common phobias can be dealt with by simply avoiding the feared object, and people who suffer from specific phobias usually do not consult professionals for help. When they do consult professionals for help, it is usually because they cannot avoid the feared situation or object or they have become obsessed with their fear and find it difficult to stop thinking about it. In this latter situation, it is sometimes difficult to distinguish phobia from obsessive-compulsive disorder. The age of onset is variable but usually begins in childhood. Phobias that do not disappear by adulthood, without treatment, usually persist throughout life.

Many specific phobias can be treated effectively with exposure therapy. In this section, treatment for several specific fears commonly seen in our practices are described. These fears include fear of heights, flying, insects, snakes, and other animals; contamination by dirt and germs; driving an automobile; and dental and medical procedures. Very unusual phobias that involve fears of objects that have not the remotest possibility of danger are rare and, when they are encountered, are usually found in psychotics.

Heights

We began this book by discusssing Goethe's fear of heights and his successful self-treatment through *in vivo* exposure. Fear of high places is one of man's most common phobias. For most people, however, fear of heights rarely interferes markedly with their lives—they simply avoid heights. People who fear heights generally feel safe in high places if they are surrounded by walls or enclosed in some way. Many feel safe if there is a railing or something solid to hold on to while they look down. Some people, for instance, will experience anxiety when looking out windows of tall buildings only if there is no sill or side wall within reaching distance.

People tend to consult therapists when severe height phobias cause them to feel anxious even in high, enclosed spaces and/or when such phobias interfere with daily functioning. For example, a client might find it necessary to undergo therapy for fear of traveling over high bridges.

In order to create a relevant flooding scene, the therapist must be able to identify the stimuli that induce the fear. Often the fear is specific to only one situation. People who are afraid of traveling over bridges may have no fear of looking out windows on the top floors of tall buildings and vice versa. Besides determining the stimulus situation, it is also necessary to understand what behavioral outcome the client may be anticipating. For example, why is the client afraid to traverse a tall bridge? Does he or she think that the bridge may collapse? Are they afraid that they might jump? Individuals who fear heights often have a fear that they will lose control and feel a compulsion to jump. These response elements should be included in the imaginal scenes presented to the client.

In treating fear of heights, it is important to encourage clients to explore and expose themselves to all aspects of the feared situation for as long as it takes for them to feel comfortable. If the fear involves looking out windows, clients are encouraged to look out the window, to look down, and to look up and try to observe all aspects of the environment. If they start to panic, they may be allowed to move away from the window for a brief interval, but then must immediately move up closer again. The client repeats the process for as many times as it takes in order to feel relatively comfortable while standing close to a window. Allowing the client to avoid the fear cue during all-out panic appears to reduce exposure time. In reality, extreme panic may actually interfere with the clients' ability to perceive or expose themselves to the fear cues. The client who fears traveling over bridges may be encouraged to start by walking rather than driving over the bridge. The client is then able to move back and forth (up and down) over the bridge in response to panic. Height phobics are encouraged to continue in the feared situation for as long as possible, but when they end the session, it should be at a point where they feel calmer and are able to express some measure of control or success.

We usually encourage clients to go through flooding first in imagination. Subsequent *in vivo* trials can be carried out either with the therapist, as homework, or both. Which procedure to use is a clinical decision. Clients who are willing to try it on their own and who have a significant other who will support them when they do their homework will often be successful without any direct therapist involvement in the *in vivo* aspect of treatment. If they are not successful with the procedure, the therapist may find it necessary to have several direct *in vivo* sessions.

An imaginal flooding scene for fear of heights might go as follows:

> You are approaching the tall bridge on foot and, as you come up to the foot of the bridge, it looks as if it climbs right into the sky. See it. It does not appear particularly stable. You notice the familiar feeling that you get when anticipating going over a high bridge. As you start walking over the bridge, notice everything. You see the steel girders. As you walk, you look down over the bridge and see the water. It occurs to you that the bridge could collapse. Feel the tension. So you move back down the bridge to a more comfortable position, closer to the foot. Feeling the anxiety reduce you again start walking up the bridge.

Case Study

Mrs. C., a 57-year-old nurse specialist, had been afraid of heights all her life. While attending a meeting on the 30th floor of the convention hotel, she had an "accidental" look out the window. At this point, she panicked and ran for the elevator. About halfway down to the first floor, the elevator stuck between floors and stalled for several minutes. This increased her panic. She was unable to return to the meeting after finally making it to the first floor. Mrs. C. consulted one of us several weeks after the convention, complaining that she was now having trouble even remaining in her office on the third floor of the hospital. Furthermore, she was unable to ride the elevator above the fourth floor.

Past history was unremarkable. The patient reported that she had always been afraid of high places, but this was the first time that she had been unable to cope with her fear inside a building. In the past, she had been afraid to climb a ladder or look out an open window above the third story, but had felt relatively safe inside a building if the windows were closed. However, she had always avoided looking out windows above the third story. She had no other significant fear nor was there any evidence of any other psychopathology.

More specific questions revealed that her fear centered on the fantasy that she might lose control and jump or fall through the open window. The elevator fear was based on the thought/image that the cables would snap and she would fall to her death or suffer serious injury. The patient also admitted to one rather bizarre fantasy involving a fear that the building would fall over "throwing" her out the window.

Flooding was both imaginal and *in vivo*. Implosive scenes centering on her fear of loss of control were also used. The scene, which included guilt and punishment cues, focused on the fear that she might purposely jump. *In vivo* flooding was graded because the client refused to start "at the top." Mrs. C. agreed to start on the third floor and to look out the window as long as the therapist held onto her hands. She further agreed to move up each succeeding floor only after becoming comfortable on the floor she was on. During *in vivo* exposure, Mrs. C. was instructed to walk to the window, look out and down and then move back. She was to continue this procedure until she could look out without experiencing significant anxiety and without holding onto the therapist's hands. During the first two 1½-hour sessions, she was unable to move to the fourth floor. By the third session, she did consent to go up one more story. Flooding went rapidly from that point. After three more sessions, she was comfortable looking out the tenth story window. Her relatively new elevator phobia was treated by using homework contracts to ride elevators at least four times per day. Thought-stopping was suggested to help control her imaginal fantasies of catastrophy (e.g., building falling over; elevator cable snapping). Therapy consisted of two imaginal flooding scenes, one implosive scene, and four *in vivo* sessions plus homework over a four week period.

Almost all height phobics that we have treated have had catastrophic fantasies. We feel that it is important and necessary to work with these fantasies in imagination and sometimes to use thought-stopping techniques. These fantasies often fit with actual experiences. For instance, when this patient became frightened, she would often feel faint, as if she were about to fall. Her fantasy that the building might fall enhanced this feeling, and both visual and proprioceptive feedback gave her the feeling that the building was actually tipping over. By having her yell "stop" to her fantasies during the *in vivo* session, while at the same time having her pay close attention to her bodily sensations, she was able to extinguish her anxiety symptoms. Implosive therapy for this case had an effect similar to paradoxical intention. As a result of the one implosive session, Mrs. C. saw the humor in her rather bizzare fantasy. She had never engaged in these fantasies when not being threatened by her fear of heights, and at those times the humor and the absurdity of the fantasies were not appreciated.

Flying

Most people have experienced some anxiety when flying in commercial airplanes. The fear is not totally irrational; the plane could crash. Yet for most flying phobics, the feeling that they have given up *control* is the most significant component of this phobia. To be completely at the mercy of other people in a situation where their miscalculation may cause you injury or death can be frightening, especially for individuals who feel the need to stay in rigid control of their lives. Many executives who feel most comfortable when they are in charge are the very people who must fly frequently. During the flight, fear stimulated by extraneous and erratic movements of the airplane leave the phobic with a sense that the pilot is losing control. To control the fear of flying many people use drugs, especially alcohol, and thus avoid the situation by clouding their sensation and perception. They often close their eyes, avoid looking out the window, and may imagine that they are someplace else. While such strategies may bring about an immediate, partial reduction in anxiety, they also serve to shelter the phobic from exposure to the feared cues. Excessive use of alcohol may be especially significant as a means of insulating the flying phobic from any positive effects that repeated exposure may have on his or her anxiety.

Treatment using *in vivo* flooding trials is best carried out in group programs that have the cooperation of the airline. However, individual therapists can successfully treat the fear of flying by a combination of instructions, flooding in imagination, and *in vivo* homework. Imaginal flooding of a bumpy flight can be followed by assigning homework to take a flight. Clients are instructed not to drink before the trip. They are also strongly encouraged to talk to the pilot about navigation, handling of the plane, and safety. It may also be helpful for the client to charter a ride in a small airplane with an instructor who can answer on-the-spot questions about the various movements of the aircraft. Most importantly, during this flight, clients are instructed not to avoid the sensations they are experiencing and the stimuli around them, but rather to explore the environment and to "go with" the experience. They may also find it helpful to use a paradoxical approach by trying to increase or emphasize the experience or to make it worse, if possible.

Another technique helpful to some flying phobics is to have them imagine that they are flying the plane during the time when turbulance jostles the plane and/or during take-off and landing. This may temporarily reduce the anxiety about loss of control but the client will continue to experience the stimuli that set off the anxiety such as movements or changes in noise level.

Case Study

Mr. J., a 41-year-old executive for a computer company, consulted us for his fear of flying after being offered a promotion that would require him to travel extensively by air. The client reported that he had always been afraid to fly. He could not recall any specific incident, such as an emergency landing or accident, that would account for his fears. When it was imperative that he fly, he would consume several ounces of alcohol before boarding and also drink during the flight. He preferred an aisle seat and was made anxious by any unusual movements or noises. Anxiety was greatest during landings. Mr. J. noted that, although the flight itself was bad enough, he made himself miserable by constantly thinking about the trip for three to four days prior to his departure. The patient was considering turning down the promotion because of his fear. Mr. J. reported no other fears or significant pathology. His catastrophic fantasy was that the plane would start losing altitude and that he would then know that he was going to die soon. He reported always feeling trapped while in the air. There were four components to treatment: (1) flooding in imagination, (2) education, (3) *in vivo* flooding, and (4) catastrophic thought-stopping.

Flooding in imagination was primarily for rehearsal or instructional purposes. Many of the cues that set off anxiety in a flying phobic are movement and/or kinesthetic and are difficult to imitate in fantasy. During the flooding scene, the client was directed to focus on a variety of cues that made him anxious, such as change in noise level or bumpiness. The educational phase of therapy involved having the client go to a local noncommercial airport and talk to a flight instructor about the realistic dangers of flying. *In vivo* flooding was accomplished in two phases: (1) taking a flight with a flight instructor in a small airplane and (2) taking a commercial flight.

During the *in vivo* commercial flight the client was instructed to sit in the window seat and not to drink either before or during the flight. He was to be aware of the various kinesthetic and visual cues that produced anxiety, and to control catastrophic thinking by "yelling" stop to himself and snapping a rubber band worn around his wrist. One year following treatment, Mr. J. was flying routinely with little or no anxiety.

Insects, Snakes, and Other Small Animals

As already noted, many analogue studies on the treatment of fear have shown that both graded and nongraded exposure techniques are effective in treating small animal fears. Most of these studies have been carried out using volunteer college students as subjects. Unfortunately, clients who consult professionals for such fears have little in common with volunteers who rate themselves as having strong fears of snakes or insects. At least 3 characteristics distinguish the analogue subject from the client. First, the client not only has a fear of small animals, but also ruminates about it much of the time. This obsessional quality is usually not found in analogue subjects.

Second, clients who worry about their fears usually suffer from a loss of self-esteem. They feel that, because they have the fear, they are weak and shameful. Analogue subjects do not usually feel this way, and are content simply to avoid the animal that they fear. Third, clients are often involved in situations that make it impossible for them to avoid the feared animal. One woman, who was treated in our clinic, had become so afraid of snakes that she would panic even at the sight of a picture of one and refused to walk on the grass or go into wooded areas. Treatment involved graded exposure because the client declined direct flooding. Imaginal exposure was used first, since she would not look at pictures of snakes. As with almost any severe phobia, secondary gain or spurious reinforcement had to be considered. In this case, the client's husband liked to fish and hunt, and he had always wanted to take his wife with him on these activities. The client, however, did not care for either sport and would not have wished to accompany her husband, even if she had no fear of snakes. Her phobia gave her a good "excuse" for not going.

Contamination

Probably the most difficult specific fear to treat with flooding are contamination fears. Here the obsessional aspect is present most clearly. Sometimes the fear is highly circumscribed and pertains to a specific place or type of contamination, but is usually generalized to anything that the client perceives as "dirty." Often these types of fears, especially if they are generalized, are driven by guilt which makes it helpful to include implosive scenes aimed at guilt cues and early life guilt experiences (usually centering around sex and aggression). Sometimes exposure can be a slow process, since most patients refuse to enter highly contaminated places or handle dirty objects. Often patients will participate in handling contaminated objects in the therapist's office but will not follow through with homework. Response prevention or stopping the client from decontaminating by using some ablution ritual is also part of the therapeutic procedure for contamination fears. This may necessitate preventing ablution for a short time after contamination and slowly increasing the length of time the patient remains contaminated. The more obsessional the client becomes about his or her contamination fear, the more likely the phobia should be subsumed under the general category of obsessive-compulsive disorder.

Case Study

Taken from Shipley and Boudewyns (1979), this case study illustrates the use of rapid *in vivo* exposure to treat a hospitalized patient with a 30-year history of severe contamination fears. Mrs. M. feared contamination by rats and rat feces. As a result of this fear, she scrubbed her hands 30 to 40 times a day (contributing to a severe eczema), used tissue to flush the toilet, and never touched the bottom of her shoes. A diagnostic interview revealed a shy, nonassertive woman with high generalized anxiety. Depression and somatic complaints were also present but appeared secondary to the neurotic fears. There were no signs of psychosis. It was explained to her how fears might be learned and the necessity of exposure to effect their reduction. It was also pointed out that each time she washed her hands out of fear, the resulting relief from fear strengthened her hand-washing habit. When she felt her hands becoming contaminated, she feared that she would become sick and die. As a result, she would be anxious and agitated. Upon scrubbing her hands, there was an immediate reduction in fear and, notably, she did not die. Compulsive habits like this are difficult to break because they work for the patient by effecting an immediate reduction in anxiety. The therapist's task is to get the patient to forgo the symptoms (hand washing) in order to learn that the feared consequence (death) will not materialize.

Mrs. M. was instructed to touch the bottom of her shoe. She did so almost automatically but then became terror-struck and started to pull her hand away. (She later rated her fear on a 0–100 scale as 150!) We strongly encouraged her to keep her hand on her shoe and rub even more of her hand across the sole. She was highly fearful and seemed to have trouble focusing on what we were saying but did as instructed. After about 5 minutes, we had her rub the sole of her other shoe with the other hand. After about 15 minutes of such exposure to her "rat contaminated" shoes, Mrs. M. was allowed to stop. She reported a very strong urge to wash her hands as she was feeling very dirty and unclean. We encouraged her to tolerate the feeling of contamination for another three hours before washing. We also agreed she would attempt to keep her hand washing to five times or less per day (response prevention).

In a session three days later, Mrs. M. reported that she had only washed her hands two to six times per day. But, since touching her shoes, she felt dirty and reported her "stomach feels like it has a hole in it." She experienced chest pains, difficulty sleeping, and generalized fearfulness. In addition, the role of hand washing in controlling guilt was revealed in her feeling "like I did something wrong." She was given support and reminded that it was expected that exposure to the "contaminated" objects would initially result in increased fear but that if she could continue to avoid washing, the fear and physical discomfort would gradually decline. She was praised for her low frequency of hand washing and instructed to keep her hand washing at or below three times per day.

By the fifth session, just seven days after she first touched the soles of her shoes, she reported much less anxiety and physical discomfort. She had washed her hands out of fear only once in two days. She was given a weekend pass and later reported washing her hands only one to two times per day while at home.

Further treatment for this patient included assertion training, imagining the feared consequences of rat contamination (implosion), training in progressive muscle relaxation, and treatment for her three-pack per day smoking habit. The contamination fear, however, had already been largely resolved.

Case Study

The following case illustrates the use of implosive scenes and *in vivo* exposure in a complicated contamination phobia. Mrs. B., a 48-year-old married woman, complained that her life had been irreparably ruined by her fear of poisons. Ten years ago, her husband had put Drano into a stopped-up drain. Mrs. B. became obsessed with the idea that the Drano was poison and that anything it touched would be contaminated. Mrs. B. suffered from severe glaucoma in both eyes and the Drano fear soon generalized to the eye drops she was supposed to put into her eyes. Because of this, she avoided using the medication and washed her hands excessively after she did use it. She also feared that she would inadvertently harm or kill people by touching them with her contaminated hands or clothes, by choking them, or by running over them with her car. Frequently while driving, she would get the idea that she had run over someone and would feel compelled to retrace her driving route to reassure herself. Similarly, if she sent a get-well card to someone in the hospital, she would later fear that the card was contaminated by her (from the Drano or eye drops) and that the person had died as a result. She would urge her husband to phone and confirm that the person was all right.

On interview, Mrs. B. presented as a passive, overly deferential woman with high moral values. Her MMPI profile was highly elevated and suggested strong subjective distress (depression and anxiety), extreme anger, passive aggressive behavior, distrustfulness, family and marital discord, and fears of loss of control. She had had multiple psychiatric hospitalizations over the past 10 years and carried a diagnosis of chronic undifferentiated schizophrenia. Past treatment included medication with Thorazine, electroconvulsive therapy, insulin therapy and insight-oriented psychotherapy. Despite the past diagnosis of schizophrenia, on interview there was no evidence of thought disorder and she made affective contact with the examiner.

Treatment was on a once a week outpatient basis and used a combination of fantasy exposure and *in vivo* exposure. Since Mrs. B. lived over three hours away from the clinic, the *in vivo* exposure was accomplished through homework assignments and by having her bring contaminated objects with her to therapy sessions. In order to bring a contaminated object to therapy, she had her husband place it in a plastic garbage bag.

In the second treatment session, a list was made of specific objects that Mrs. B. avoided because she feared they were contaminated. Prominantly included on the list were wastebaskets, her husband's shoes (believed to be contaminated by Drano), and certain areas of her kitchen and bathroom (again thought to be contaminated by Drano and/or eye drops). Mrs. B. completely avoided the "contaminated" den where her husband spent much of his time. In the third session, a neutral imagery scene showed that Mrs. B. had good imaging ability. This was followed by an implosive scene in which she was asked to picture herself sitting in the Drano-contaminated chair in her den. This scene led to high anxiety (rated 100 on a 0–100 anxiety scale). Mrs. B. was asked to expose herself to the scene two times each day as homework.

In the fourth session, Mrs. B. reported accomplishing her homework once a day and rated her anxiety level during these scenes at 50. An implosive therapy scene was presented in which she again imagined sitting in the contaminated recliner and experienced the feelings of contamination and anxiety. She then "killed" various people, primarily people she regarded with some ambivalence, by touching them with her contaminated body. She rated this scene at 75, and it was assigned as homework. In the fifth session she reported again doing the homework once per day, with decreasing anxiety over the course of the week. She expressed anger towards her husband in a more direct fashion than she had done previously. No scene was accomplished during the session but she was asked to imagine as homework being contaminated by Drano and again killing people by touching them. She was also asked to bring to the next session the pair of her husband's shoes which she viewed as the most contaminated.

In session 6, she brought in the shoes. In this session, she was forcefully but empathetically encouraged to touch the contaminated shoes. This, of course, led to very high fear, but Mrs. B. was continually encouraged to remain in contact with the contaminated shoes, to touch every surface with both hands, and to touch her hands to other parts of her body and clothes. After 30 minutes, an observed reduction in her level of distress occurred and she was allowed to put the shoes down. She agreed not to wash, shower, or change clothes for the next five hours, despite strong feelings of contamination. Further, she was to continue practicing her homework implosive therapy scenes. In session 7, she was again exposed *in vivo* to her husband's shoes and she was assigned the homework of touching a wastebasket for four 1-hour sessions and was to wait 2 hours thereafter before washing. Additionally, to maintain her gains with her husband's shoes, she was instructed to touch the shoes for at least five minutes each day, also without washing afterwards.

In session 8, she reported successfully accomplishing the homework assignments, although she was terrified and cried a lot. Her fears of the wastebaskets decreased from 100 to 40 on the anxiety scale. The shoes elicited very little anxiety for her and she reported they were "sort of becoming like old friends." The homework assignment involved her briefly touching the wastebasket each day and exposing herself to a cushion of her husband's contaminated chair, with further instructions to bring in some very contaminated newspapers from the den for the next session.

Sessions 9 and 10 continued this basic *in vivo* strategy with the additional instructions that, despite her feeling contaminated and capable of killing people by touching them, she was to touch as many people during the day as possible. For sessions 11 and 12, she brought in her eye drops and was asked to place them in her hands and to rub them all over while agreeing not to wash for several hours thereafter.

Sessions 13, 14, and 15 dealt with her fears that she would express her anger by touching and killing someone with her contaminated hands or body. She was convinced to put a drop of her eye medication on her hands prior to cooking or entering the kitchen. Then she was to bake something and bring it for the therapist's consumption. (Being a conservative sort, the therapist first had the patient check with her local pharmacist to reassure patient and therapist that nothing in the eye drops was actually harmful.) At this point, Mrs. B. had regained the run of her house, was able to put her eye drops in without fear or excessive hand washing, and had stopped her checking rituals to see if she had killed someone. She was most happy with her progress but was still experiencing much marital discord. Marital therapy followed with only moderate success. At the time of this writing, over one year following therapy termination, Mrs. B. continues to be largely free of contamination fears. She does, however, occasionally acquire a new contamination fear. For example, she has feared rat poison and bug sprays used on trees. In each case, she has treated these fears before they gained momentum by using *in vivo* exposure. The marriage, however, continues to be problematic.

Automobile Driving

Fear of driving usually begins with an incident in which the client has an anxiety-provoking experience while driving a car. This can be anything from an accident to an anxiety attack while, but unrelated to, driving. Often that person may find it more difficult to drive on the logic that he or she will panic and pass out and have an accident. These catastrophic thoughts of the feared event may quickly bring on an anxiety attack that redintegrates the earlier experience that reinforces the fear. Driving phobics often describe themselves as "frozen" to the steering wheel and feeling like they cannot manipulate the floor pedals. As the fear persists, most limit their driving to areas of little traffic and avoid high speed roads, bridges, and other areas where driving is more difficult. Eventually, they may give up driving altogether.

Instruction in panic control is generally the first phase of treatment. Panic control provides clients with an alternative to avoidance behavior as a means of dealing with extreme anxiety. If clients feel a panic attack is imminent and they are unable to control it, they are instructed to pull off the road and relax, but then to return to the feared situation as soon as possible. Therapists should emphasize the importance of getting back on the road after a bad experience and that the client should never totally leave the feared situation in a panic. To do so will only increase fear through the reinforcement of anxiety reduction and through loss of self-confidence.

Treatment is frequently *in vivo.* Clients are first encouraged to drive with the therapist. *In vivo* flooding with the therapist present, however, does not ordinarily extinguish anxiety. Most driving phobics experience little anxiety when the therapist is in the car with them. However, the practice with the therapist instructs the client in how to carry out homework assignments. The homework contracts encourage the client to drive a specific amount each day. The homework provides continued exposure to the driving situation which is the key element in treatment.

Case Study

Mrs. K. was a 33-year-old housewife and part-time waitress whose only goal of therapy was to be able to drive her car without anxiety. She had been anxious about driving for the past eight years but had stopped driving altogether after an incident in which she experienced a severe panic attack while driving alone. At that time, the client pulled off the road, left the car, called her father and had him take her home. She decided to stop driving on the assumption that future attacks could lead to a loss of control and cause her to have an accident. She also found the panic attacks in and of themselves extremly aversive and simply wished to avoid that experience altogether.

Mrs. K. was typical of most driving phobics in that her fear was not equal in all driving situations. Heavy traffic made it more difficult for her to pull off the road and thus increased her anxiety, which in turn would increase the likelihood that she would panic. This "fear cycle," common to many phobias, was the basis of Mrs. K.'s problem. Therapy was carried out in three phases: (1) instruction in panic control, (2) *in vivo* flooding, and (3) homework.

Observation revealed that, while driving, Mrs. K. remained extremely alert to both her own anxiety level and the traffic situation. If traffic became heavy or if she felt "trapped" on the road, she reported that she would tighten up, grip the wheel hard and sit up close to the windshield. She was instructed to counter this anxiety response by deep breathing exercises and muscle relaxation. If a panic attack seemed imminent, Mrs. K. was told to pull off to the side of the road as soon as possible, take two deep breaths and then engage in progressive muscle relaxation. Since muscle tension was an important component in this woman's anxiety, she was trained in Bernstein and Borkovec's (1973) tension release exercises.

Initially, Mrs. K. was asked to drive at least one-half hour per day, even if she had no place to go. She was also encouraged *not* to avoid heavy traffic, to keep a log of her driving time, and to note her feelings before, during, and after driving. Mrs. K. was highly motivated and after two weeks of homework reported that she was able to drive alone with only minor discomfort. She is still being followed at this writing.

Often fear of driving is one component of a more complex problem. It may be associated with claustrophobia, fear of loss of control, agoraphobia, or posttraumatic stress syndrome. In such cases, the driving fear is treated in the larger context. As illustrated in the case discussed below, treatment may involve fantasy implosive therapy with no *in vivo* exposure. Frequently, however, *in vivo* exposure is still necessary following implosion to the hypothesized stimuli complex.

Case Study

A 26-year-old lawyer presented with complaints of recurrent anxiety attacks with tingling in his left arm, heart palpitations, and depersonalization. The attacks might occur at any time but were most likely to occur when the patient was driving or while pleading a case in court. Numerous extensive medical work-ups were negative. The patient appeared tense and depressed and reported that he had decided to give up the practice of law.

In attempting to determine the stimuli eliciting the anxiety attacks, the therapist explored in detail the situations present during various individual anxiety attacks while searching for commonalities. The first anxiety attack, which occurred in court on a Wednesday, took place during what the patient knew was, or should have been, a simple case. He was defending a teenager in a civil suit, but knew he was going to wrongly lose this suit. All he had to do was to ask witnesses a few questions and get the expected answers and then wait for the expected verdict. Later, anxiety attacks were most likely to occur on Wednesday afternoons when the patient handled routine juvenile court cases in which his client was pleading guilty. These cases were frequently less demanding than cases he handled during the rest of the week, yet were associated with the anxiety attacks.

The anxiety attacks that occurred while driving were also said to be unpredictable and not associated with anything in particular. However, detailed questioning about individual anxiety attacks revealed that they were most likely to occur when it was raining or when the pavement was wet following a rain. Also, if he was feeling hurried or had missed a turn or was otherwise not in full control, anxiety was more likely.

The answer to the diagnostic riddle came when the therapist asked about past traumatic events—illnesses, accidents, and fights. The client revealed that at age 15 he was in an auto accident in which he had been driving and his best friend had been killed. When the accident occurred, the pavement was wet and the patient had missed a turn in the road. The car crashed into an oncoming car, killing his friend who was riding in the front seat next to him. The patient admitted to some guilt in that in trying to avoid the oncoming car, he turned the wheel such that the right side of the car and his friend took the full impact of the crash. He was left-handed and it was this hand and arm that turned the wheel causing, in his view, his friend's death. Some years later, the friend's family brought suit against the patient and, following a jury trial, the patient was found guilty and ordered to pay a cash award. The patient felt this was an injustice.

The traumatic events of the car accident and the jury trial had obvious similarities to the situations currently leading to the anxiety attacks. Attacks while driving occurred when the stimulus situation resembled that of the car accident (wet pavement, missing a turn). Attacks in the court room occurred in situations similar to his own traumatic court room experience as a teenager. Exploration of recurrent dreams tended to confirm the importance of these events in the patient's symptoms. The patient dreamed of seeing his best friend alive and saying that he was only smashed up. The patient says, "I hope you aren't mad at me" and his friend replys, "God no, it wasn't your fault; the other guy was going 80 miles an hour."

The accident caused discord between the patient and his friends, with many expressing feelings that the patient was a callous rich kid. Some years after the accident, he had a very traumatic fist fight with a former friend who thought him a killer. Further complicating the patient's reaction to this trauma was the fact that his friend's mother had always been like a loving mother to him, whereas his own mother had been cold, rejecting, and neurotic.

Other problems involved extreme anger toward authority figures, strong fears of failure, illness and death, and fears of homosexuality. He had also recently become impotent. The first implosive therapy scene, however, dealt with the car accident. The scene replayed the accident, adding only the guilt cues to the actual events; later scenes in the courtroom added guilt and anger cues. Some repetition has been removed to shorten the narrative but the reader should remember that repetition is an essential ingredient for the extinction of negative emotion.

T. You're in your car on your way back to the city. Jack is next to you. You are in a hurry, driving fast. You decide to take the shortcut home. You are driving very fast. You can see the lane markers changing before your eyes, the trees on both sides of the road. You feel the steering wheel in your left hand. Put your hand out now as if it's resting on the wheel. The pavement is wet and you are just rounding the curve now, onto the road to take a shortcut and you feel yourself being pulled into the wrong lane. You miss the turn and you drift into the wrong lane. Do you see that?

C. Yes.

T. There is a car coming head-on. You see that car and you realize there is no way to escape. You see the hills on both sides of the curve and there is no way out and the car is right on top of you now and you think, "I don't want to die. I don't want to die. I would rather have Jack dead. Yes, Jack should die," and so you swerve to the left. You feel your left hand and arm pulling down that wheel. That's right. Pull down on that wheel now and you swerve to the left to get yourself out of danger and you feel the tinglingness in your left arm as you do that. Can you feel that?

C. Yes, my arm is all tingling.

T. And you feel that tinglingness and your heart is racing and you are in a cold sweat. You can feel the tightness across your chest, the tinglingness in your left arm and you see that car coming at you, coming at Jack's side now and then there's a big crash. And you watch as the metal goes into Jack like a knife and you know that you have killed him. You have killed him. It's your fault. You pulled down with your left hand on that steering wheel so that he would get the impact and you could save yourself. You missed the curve, didn't you? See that again now. See that again—it's wet, the pavement is wet. You are rounding the curve. You are going into the other lane now. The car is coming, it's coming right for you. Pull down on that wheel and feel those sensations in your arm, feel them. That's right! That's right! Feel them and feel the tension and the anxiety and the fear and feel and know that you are doing this so that you can live. You are sacrificing your best friend and then crash!! CRASH!! And the metal is going through him. You feel the impact yourself and you see that he is dying now. The next thing you know you are sitting by the side of the road and the other driver is saying, "You were in my lane, you were in my lane!" And you are saying, "I'm allergic to penicillin, I'm allergic to penicillin!" And the other driver says, "You killed that other boy. You killed him." And you say "I'm allergic to penicillin." You're in the ambulance now and you hear the siren and Jack is beside you and you hear the driver and the attendant talking and they say "one is dead. He is dead. He was killed by that little rich kid, that little rich kid out in the car." Later, after you recover, you have that fight with Bob with your friends all watching and calling you all those terrible names. See Bob's angry face glaring at you. He knows you killed his friend, doesn't he? He knows you're responsible. He knows you killed him and he hits you and you feel the pain as he hits you again and again and again. And you feel also the pain of all your friends looking on and knowing that you are a flippant killer who actually had no love for Jack, who killed him, and you feel the pain of the blows and you feel the pain of the hate of your friends but later remember that Jack's mother loves you. You remember what she said after the crash; you see her face now, and she is saying, "Don't ever worry. I will always love you like my own son," and you feel secure in that and happy because, unlike your own mother, Jack's mother loves you and she forgives you and she bears no grudge. "Don't every worry, I will always love you like my own son." But then Bob talks to her and convinces her that you killed her son in cold blood and she decides to get her revenge, doesn't she? She brings suit against you for killing her son in cold blood. It's like you have been betrayed and no one loves you and they all hate you and they all think you are a killer. See yourself in the courtroom. There is the judge sitting up there high above you and the jury, and Bob and Jack's parents are there. Jack's brother who hates you so and . . . *(the courtroom scene continues with the patient eventually found guilty and experiencing the anxiety, guilt, and anger engendered by that verdict).**

The above scene was presented in each of the next three therapy sessions with the client practicing it at home two to three times daily. The client never again experienced an anxiety attack or a nightmare regarding these events. Four additional sessions dealt with the fear of failure (primarily failure in his private law practice), the remaining anger toward his parents and other authority figures, and with the fears of homosexuality related to a hypothesized Oedipal situation. With these latter scenes, the impotence was resolved and he was more comfortable in his legal practice. Prior to therapy, the neurotic triad on the MMPI (hypochondriasis, depression, and hysteria) was above normal limits. Following therapy, the client's profile was entirely within normal limits. A 6-month follow-up showed no recurrence of symptoms.

Fear of Dental Procedures

In advanced societies, the fear of going to the dentist may be even more common than the fear of snakes. The etiology of the fear usually involves aversive childhood experiences with the dentist. The case described below demonstrates how flooding and implosive therapy can be used with a severe dental fear.

CASE STUDY

Donald, a 25-year-old unmarried welder, was admitted to an inpatient psychiatric unit complaining of depression and anxiety. He had a history of criminal behavior, a spotty work record, lacked social and academic skills, and was unemployed. A milieu therapy program was developed to work on these problems. It was also suggested that he join a remedial reading class and obtain further technical training as a welder.

*Again, the supportive client therapist interaction that followed this scene have been omitted.

After entering the program, it was discovered that Donald also had a specific fear of dentists and dental offices. His teeth were in a severe state of decay, but his fear had kept him from consulting a dentist since the age of seven. He stated that if he even attempted to enter a dentist's office he would feel nauseated and would gag and vomit.

The fear appeared to stem from a frightening childhood experience when Donald had one of his teeth pulled by what he described as a "mean and ugly dentist." Donald agreed to try flooding to overcome his fear. The therapy consisted of: (1) three sessions of imaginal flooding, (2) homework, in which Donald was encouraged to go through the imaginal scene on his own, and (3) somewhat graded *in vivo* flooding procedure.

Two basic scenes were used. Both involved symptom–contingent cues. The first imaginal scene was a straightforward account of a trip to the dental service at the hospital. The scene essentially described what was to become the *in vivo* flooding program. In the other scene, he relived the trip to the "mean and ugly" dentist. Initially, Donald had difficulty remembering the details of the experience and stated that he didn't like to think about it anyway. After some encouragement and aided by hypnosis, he was able to remember the experience in surprising detail. Therapy consisted of guiding his imagery while he recalled the frightening experience. Donald's transcript of his trip to the dentist is interesting because of the detailed manner in which he recalled the event. His recall was not dissimilar to the way some veterans remember dramatic war experiences under hypnosis, although he did not experience the other symptoms of post-traumatic stress syndrome described earlier in this chapter.*

T. OK. Donald, now I want you to close your eyes and imagine when you were seven years old. It was the morning that you went to have your tooth pulled at the dentist's office. You recall it very clearly now. You are starting to walk out the door. Your mother has given you a note with instructions on how to get to the dentist and you are going to walk there all by yourself. You start to feel some of the anxiety already. You have never had an experience with the dentist but you have heard others talk about it and you know that your tooth hurts. OK.? Begin.

C. Yeah. I remember walking out the door and going down the street. I'm thinking about I *have* to go to the dentist. I walk on down to a busy street. I believe it was called K-K street; and as I start down the street, I see the soda shop on my left. I go into the soda shop and sit down and order a soda.

T. What kind of soda?

C. Coke.

T. OK. See that Coke now. You are sitting there at the counter drinking your

*For scenes that involve recalling anxiety-producing past events, the therapist can remain relatively passive until the client shows an increase in anxiety or emotionality. At that point, the therapist should give instructions to slow down and to relive the past experience as vividly as possible.

Coke trying to avoid going to the dentist. Trying to take just a little more time before you go to the dentist.

C. Well, yeah. Then I started talking to a friend and she told me about the dentist, and I remember her saying that she had gone to the dentist and it didn't seem to bother her at all. I felt better about it then. Anyway, I'm sitting there for a while and I feel that I should get going, but I wait just a little bit longer. I'm waiting for my check anyway. But my check came right away and it wouldn't have bothered me if it had taken her a little longer to figure out how much the bill was. So then I got off of the stool and went out the drugstore and went across the street to the smokeshop. I remember standing there at the smokeshop looking at all the pipes and things.

T. Can you smell that smokeshop, too?

C. No. I didn't go in. I was just looking at the pipes and things. I just thought they looked neat. I wasn't smoking then.

T. Well, you've got to go the dentist. You can't avoid going to the dentist.

C. Yeah. Well, I walked kind of slow but I finally got to the dentist and his office was upstairs. I remember seeing the stairway and I was looking at the stairway and I counted the stairs as I went up. I remember that there was exactly 32 stairs. I got up to the second floor and I started talking to a maid there. I said to her, "I have to go to Dr. A.'s office." She showed me the way. Well, when I got to Dr. A.'s office there was a note on the door, and I couldn't read it, so I got the maid to read it. She said that I had to go to another doctor, Dr. B., down the hall because Dr. A. was out of town that day and this other doctor was taking his cases. So I walked down the hall and went into Dr. B.'s office and talked to the nurse there. I looked around awhile and told her who I was and what my problem was. She told me to sit down and she would call me when Dr. B. was ready to see me.

T. OK. Can you see the room there? Try to smell all that medicine smell that you talked about. Imagine as clearly as possible.

C. Yeah. I can see it. It really, ew, gives me the creeps to think about it. I can feel myself starting to get anxious. *(Client sits up in his chair and grabs the sides tighter)*

T. OK. Now I want you to imagine this as clearly as possible. The nurse calls you.

C. Yeah. I can hear her.

T. OK. Now you go into the dentist's office. OK. What happened from there?

C. OK. Well, he puts me on this board—on this chair. He made me lay back in the chair. I looked at him and he kind of smiled and it didn't look like it was bothering him at all. And he said, "Now sit back, this won't hurt." So I sat back and he got out these kind of plier-like things. Not pliers but things that look like pliers. He said, "Open up." I did and he looked in and he said, "Yeah, you've got a bad one there." He took those pliers and he got hold of the tooth and he started to pull.

T. OK. Feel that pulling sensation.

C. Yeah, he pulled. And when he pulled, he pulled my whole head down and I started to cry. I said, "It hurts." He pushed me back into the chair and he said, "Shut up, and let me finish this." He pulled some more. *(Client starting to show tears in his eyes at this point.)* He kept pulling. I can feel that and I can see that. Ew. He was a mean and ugly looking dentist. It seemed like it just took him forever and it hurt so bad. Each time he pulled, I pulled down with my head and he had to push me back. Then he twisted it *(client tightens up)* and pulled it and pulled it and pulled it. Finally, it came out. Ew. I can remember the taste. I was so mad at him that I started to cry. *(Client starts to cry.)* I wanted to hit him but I knew that I couldn't, and there was blood in my mouth and he put some of this cotton-like stuff in my mouth to stop the bleeding. I sat there and I cried and he said, "Hush now, you can go on home. It's all over."

T. OK. I want you to feel that now. Feel that pulling sensation again. We're going to go through that again . . .

After three imaginal visits and homework practice, Donald evidenced a considerable reduction in anxiety to the scenes and could recount the childhood experience without obvious emotionality.

During *in vivo* flooding Donald was escorted by the therapist to the outer office of the dental service in the hospital. He was encouraged to stay there as long as possible or until he felt no anxiety. On the next day he was taken into the inside office to have his teeth X-rayed and checked. Within two weeks, he had successfully endured several visits to the dentist.

This case demonstrates a rather simple flooding of a specific fear. However, reliving the childhood experience that Donald had avoided was also a significant aspect of treatment.

This scene brought out considerable anger and depressive affect related to the fact that Donald's mother had made him go to the dentist without support. Donald's relationship with his mother was a source of difficulty for him and was later treated in family therapy.

Medical and Surgical Procedures

Fears of medical and surgical procedures are common and they are often reasonable. A large body of research indicates that patients provided with procedural and sensory information and/or shown a filmed or live model undergoing the procedure are generally less anxious than controls (Shipley, 1982). Occasionally, such fears reach phobic proportions and may prevent patients from receiving needed diagnostic and treatment procedures. Such cases can be treated with exposure therapy in much the same way as the dental phobic reviewed above. Alternatively, a flooding technique may be used in which the patient repeatedly observes the medical procedure or a video tape of the procedure until anxiety diminishes significantly. Ghose, Giddon, Shiere, and Eogels (1969), for example, had children observe their older siblings receiving dental treatment prior to their own treatment. We have prepared patients for stressful medical procedures by exposing them repeatedly to a video tape of a patient undergoing the same procedure (Shipley, Butt, Horwitz, & Farbry, 1978; Shipley, Butt, & Horwitz, 1979).

Case Study

Sharon, a 17-year-old, required an upper endoscopy examination but was terrified of the procedure. The procedure is, indeed, a stressful one involving the insertion of a 12 mm diameter scope through the mouth and throat and into the gastrointestinal tract. Air is pumped into the gut and a physician manipulates the endoscope for 15–30 minutes while viewing the GI tract. The patient is awake throughout the procedure and must cooperate. On two occasions, when entering the endoscopy area, Sharon began screaming hysterically and ran from the room. Subsequently, she was shown an explicit video tape of a patient receiving an endoscopy. During her first viewing of the tape, she displayed obvious fear by gripping her chair and breathing rapidly. By the third viewing of the tape, she appeared quite calm and exhibited a more detached intellectual interest in the procedure. The following morning she underwent the examination with minimal distress and required no sedation.

For more details on preparing patients for stressful medical/surgical procedures see Shipley (1982).

Social Phobia

Social phobia is defined as a persistent irrational fear that results in a desire to avoid situations where the person feels vulnerable to embarrassment or criticism by others. People who suffer from social phobias are afraid that in public places they will do something that will embarrass and humiliate themselves. They are constantly anticipating such humiliation and are careful to avoid situations where they might be scrutinized by others.

Social phobia should be distinguished from agoraphobia. The agoraphobic tends to be afraid of *any* public place whereas a social phobic is more specific. Social phobias include fears of urinating in public laboratories, eating in public, or writing in the presence of others. Rarely, however, does the social phobic have more than one of these types of fears. Performance anxiety is marked by a vicious cycle that is created when this irrational fear increases anxiety in the public situation that in turn impairs performance, thus giving the phobic good reason to avoid the situation in the future.

Social phobias often begin in late childhood or early adolescence. Many start with anxiety-provoking experiences while in school (e.g., performing poorly in front of a class and being criticized; forgetting lines in a school play). The disorder is chronic and may last throughout the individual's lifetime. As with any phobia, professionals are usually not consulted unless the disorder begins to interfere with the individual's life or when avoidance of the situation becomes difficult. Obsessional social phobics may consult therapists because the fear has diminished their self-esteem.

Social phobia, interpersonal anxiety, and problems with assertion can be effectively treated with exposure. The case study below demonstrates the use of these techniques with a nonassertive male with severe interpersonal anxiety that was exacerbated by interaction with anyone, especially authority figures.

Case Study

Ron, a 30-year-old married foreman for an aluminum window manufacturer was admitted with complaints of nervousness, generalized uncontrolled tremors (more pronounced in his fingers and hands), and a history of seizure-like episodes. A neurologist concluded that his symptoms were psychogenic. Psychotropic medications had no significant effect. Because his wife was about to have their first child, the family's financial situation was going to become a further source of anxiety for him if he were unable to leave the hospital and return to work promptly.

In the pretherapy interview, the patient reported that his symptoms had been pronounced for the past three or four years, although he had felt anxious and inadequate since graduation from high school. Exacerbation of symptoms coincided with the onset of his wife's pregnancy.

Ron described his early childhood as pleasant up until the age of 12 when the family bought a small farm. Here he was given "too many responsibilities." When he was unable to perform his chores adequately, his father who drank heavily, would physically punish him. No specific stimulus seemed associated with the symptoms but, considering the patient's history, it was not surprising that he disliked being put in any position of responsibility. He was also disturbed when he would see or even read about any form of violence. However, the client's immediate concerns were the embarrassment he felt when his hands "shock so much that other could see," and the fear that he might "blackout" at an unfortunate time (e.g., while driving).

Not including the two initial interview sessions, therapy consisted of twelve 45-minute sessions over a period of 3½ weeks. During this time, it was suggested to the patient that he make no effort to control his tremors. In fact, he was instructed to try to shake more when he felt episodes coming on. Although skeptical at first, the client was pleased to find that this procedure actually increased self-control over the shaking in anxiety-provoking situations. Although this suggestion is consistent with the theory that underlines flooding and implosive therapy, the reader may notice the similarity between this and Frankel's Paradoxical Intention technique.

Early scenes centered around Ron's embarrassment about his shaking. Later themes were based on his past life and emphasized aggression, counter aggression, punishment, parental rejection, and failure in positions of responsibility.

Ron did not display much affect during therapy. An increase in his anxiety was indicated by greater postural rigidity. In this case, the patient's effort at rigid control may simply have been a means that he had used in the past to keep from shaking. Each scene was repeated within each session and then assigned as homework; the scene would also be reviewed during the next session until there was a reduction in the patient's emotional response. Ron was successfully treated with implosive therapy using only imaginal scenes. Treatment sessions are described briefly below.

Session 1. During the initial interview session, Ron was asked to describe what situations were relatively more anxiety-provoking for him. One situation he described involved his carpool. He was especially anxious when it was his turn to drive. This fact was consistent with the patient's fear of failure and punishment when he was in positions of responsibility. Thus, his fear that he would have an accident while driving and be responsible for other people's injuries, or possible death, was of great concern to him. While actually driving, he would avoid his fears by driving slowly and attending to the external stimuli of the road and environment.

The imagined scene consisted of an accident in which all members of the carpool, except the client, were killed in a bloody, two-car crash. He was then punished by his family and friends. Punishment consisted of another fear, the fear of rejection and loneliness. The scene concluded with the client in solitary confinement where no one even recognized his existence. He died painfully in his cell as a lonely man. The scene ended here since the client did not have strong religious convictions about afterlife. If he had, it would have been appropriate to continue imaginal punishment in the hereafter.

Session 2. This scene's cues were similar to those in scene one, but involved situations in which the patient was put into positions of responsibility while in military service. At one point during his career, Ron had been a prison guard. This position had made him extremely anxious for two reasons: (1) he feared he would not be able to meet his responsibilities and the prisoners would escape, and (2) he was concerned about his own response should prisoners try to escape. He doubted that he would be able to shoot at them if they were to make an attempt. It was hypothesized that this fear of aggression was originally learned as the result of the punishment he received as a child. His father had routinely punished Ron's assertiveness. Ron feared that, if he engaged in violent activities, he would lose control of himself and end up being rejected and punished for his behavior. Thus, the scene stressed these very fears by having him imagine the prisoners escaping, him being punished for his irresponsibility, and his counter aggression at the authority that punished him. His violent reactions were then met by further violence on the part of the authorities and again he ended up being rejected and punished. This time he was asked to imagine being sentenced to die in a gas chamber by a punitive judge who looked like his father. A relevant fact here is that Ron was prejudiced against policemen and other law enforcement officials. These negative feelings were easily tapped with this scene.

Session 3. The scene for this session was derived from Ron's hostility toward his boss. He claimed that his boss demanded too much of him and gave him too much responsibility without sufficient remuneration. The scene centered around an argument between the patient and his boss that led to Ron being fired. At this point, the patient was asked to imagine becoming hostile and starting a fist fight that ended with him clubbing his boss to death. The scene concluded with the patient being charged with assault and again sentenced, rejected, and put to death in the gas chamber.

Session 4. The scene for session 4 centered around another symptom—contingent cue; that is, Ron's embarrassment over shaking when other people made demands on him. Ron claimed that his hands would shake most when he would reach out to accept an item offered to him by another person. Consequently, if at all possible, he would avoid such interaction. This theme encompassed a number of embarrassing situations in which the patient would shake so much that he would spill and drop things on others. He would then be ridiculed for the behavior. Hostility toward authority figures was emphasized in this scene as well.

Session 5. For session 5, two scenes were presented that involved hostile, angry responses towards familiar authority figures and some of the same cues presented in scenes one, two, and three, were reviewed. By this time, most of the symptom–contingent cues had been covered in some detail. Ron also cooperated by carrying out his homework assignments.

Sessions 6, 7, and 8. In these sessions, hypothesized cues from Ron's early life were presented. The scene centered around hypothesized arguments with his father concerning Ron's farm responsibilities when he was 12 years old. His father was pictured as drunk and abusive. Ron returned the hostility. This resulted in the patient being severely punished by his father and ostracized by his mother and the rest of the family for his aggression. The client's emotional response to this scene was strong and may have represented a core element of his problem.

Session 9. This session's scene centered around the hypothesized cues of conflict, frustration, rejection, abandonment, punishment, and physical discomfort as an infant. This did not elicit a great deal of anxiety and it was hypothesized that Ron's present conditioned fears were probably not associated with experiences before the age of 12.

Session 10. Since it could be hypothesized that the client's feelings of inadequacy and his fear of masculine authority might be rooted in his concern of not measuring up to acceptable standards of masculinity, this scene centered around homosexual cues. Ron responded with little or no anxiety to this theme so it was not pursued further.

Session 11. Since the patient was about to become a father and there was some indication that this was one of the factors that brought him into the hospital, a scene was presented in which he lost control of his anger towards his child (i.e., taking his own father's role and the child taking his role). The client responded with considerable affect.

Session 12. In the twelfth session, the scene again centered around the same cues that were presented in session 11, but also included the anger he felt towards his wife as a consequence of being rejected in favor of the child.

By the end of therapy, the tremors had dissipated considerably and disappeared entirely within two months after the last session. Also, the patient's MMPI profile, which before therapy was elevated on both scales two (Depression) and seven (Anxiety), fell within normal limits four months after the last session. At that time, Ron informed the therapist that for the first time in his life he could actually enjoy movies with violence in them. He also reported that arguments with his wife and boss were not nearly so stressful as they had been before therapy.

Public Speaking

Anxiety about making public appearances of any type can be treated by flooding in imagination but must be followed by *in vivo* homework to be effective. For performance fears, it is helpful if flooding is offered in the context of the client exploring the irrational causes of his or her fear. Role playing in the relatively safe situation of the therapist's office with a surrogate audience is also useful. If the client has little opportunity to practice public speaking, he or she may be encouraged to join the local chapter of the *Toastmaster's Club.* This is an organization that helps people develop and perfect public speaking skills.

CASE STUDY

Mrs. F., a 32-year-old social worker, had experienced public speaking fears since Jr. High School. She recalled her first trauma vividly. In the ninth grade a teacher called on her to recite a poem. When she stumbled on a word and made it sound profane, the class laughed at her and the teacher scolded her. She became so panicky about continuing that she left the room in embarrassment. From that time on, she had avoided almost all public speaking. If she were required to speak in public, her anxiety level would remain high for several days prior to the time she had to appear. We were consulted because she was considering taking a teaching position that would require her to lecture to a large class at least once per week. She felt it was imperative that she reduce her public speaking fear before she committed herself to the position. Mrs. F. complained of no other fears and there appeared to be no other significant pathology. There were four steps in this client's treatment: (1) imaginal flooding, (2) cognitive restructuring, (3) *in vivo* flooding (role playing), and (4) homework.

Imaginal flooding consisted of the scene recalling her Jr. High School experience as well as scenes imagining projected symptom–contingent cues such as lecturing to her anticipated class. The client was instructed to practice these scenes at home until anxiety diminished. The imaginal scenes generated only minimal anxiety. *In vivo* sessions involved having Mrs. F. role play several speeches for a surrogate audience. This exercise appeared to be quite anxiety provoking for her. The client was exposed to three *in vivo* therapy sessions using the surrogate audience. After each speech, the audience gave her feedback on her performance.*

Most public speaking fears are maintained because clients tell themselves that it would be terrible if their anxiety symptoms, such as their shaking legs or cracking voice, were observed by the audience. To counter this, Mrs. F. was given homework requiring her to seek out an audience and give a speech to them. Before she started speaking, however, she was told to admit to the audience that she was afraid to speak in public and that, if her voice cracked or her legs shook, they were to ignore it because it would go away. This ploy is effective but is often resisted by the client. Most feel that to admit the anxiety is to embarrassing in and of itself. Persuading the client to overcome this sensitivity is sometimes difficult, but it is an important part of this treatment.

Mrs. F. was able to take her new position. One year after treatment, however, she stated that she still felt mildly anxious during her lectures.

Urinating in Public Restrooms

Probably more common today than in previous years is the anxiety, primarily among men, associated with urinating in public toilets. The increase in this fear may be due to the fact that in today's society there is a much greater emphasis on privacy than there was previously. For instance, older army barracks had as a urinal nothing more than a long trough at which several men at a time could stand and urinate. Today, barracks are outfitted with individual, private stalls. The same is true for

*Public speaking phobics tend to overestimate how much their anxiety "shows." Accurate feedback helps increase their confidence in their ability to control outward signs of anxiety.

other public accommodations. If a fear of urinating in public starts to develop in a young boy, there is little opportunity for him to extinguish that fear. Then, on those occasions when he does encounter open urinals, he may not be able to urinate and this failure reinforces the anxiety. Soon, through the process of generalization and irrational thinking, he ends up unable to relax his bladder, regardless of the degree of privacy in the public restroom. The irrational thinking underlying the fear is that someone will enter the restroom before the client starts to urinate, see that he is unable to do so, and recognize his inadequacy. This thought increases anxiety and sympathetic activity that, of course, inhibits the parasympathetic activation necessary to relax one's bladder. In borderline personalities, this fear may also be associated with some psychosexual concerns and may involve a fear that other men in the restroom might view their inability to urinate as a lack of masculinity and confront them, or, worse yet, make a homosexual proposition. Such cases are more involved, and exposure treatment should address these issues.

Flooding as treatment for public urination fear is relatively straightforward. The client is taken to a public toilet and required to stand at the urinal with a male therapist until he finally urinates. Homework involves standing in public toilets, no matter how long it takes to urinate, while at the same time practicing a more rational thought process. Clients are instructed to say to themselves, "What do I care what others think? They can't hurt me." Homework is probably the most important part of therapy. The *in vivo* flooding with the therapist is primarily instructional. In our experience, success depends solely on how much and how often a client practices. Many clients will not allow direct flooding, but instead use a graded approach starting with relatively safe, public restrooms where few people are likely to enter. Unfortunately, "safe" and "unsafe" public restrooms are relatively discrete and separate conditions and do not lend themselves easily to the development of a desensitization hierarchy or to generalization of that hierarchy. Clients are strongly encouraged to start at the top and learn to stand there and relax their bladder.

Case Study

Mr. J. was a 26-year-old systems analyst who was referred to us by a psychiatrist. The client's inability to urinate in public toilets, especially if there was someone else in the restroom or if he could not lock the door, was inconvenient and had resulted in a diminished self-concept. He reported that he had always been sensitive about public restrooms, but the problem had become worse since his graduation from school. It was hypothesized that the fear had become more of a problem because he now worked for a company where the men's toilets were relatively large and open. Further, when he entered the men's room at work, he would often meet a friend, who would casually strike up a conversation. Mr. J. found this situation extremely difficult because he then had to go into a private stall and sit on the commode. The client was concerned that, if he continued such behavior, his friends would come to suspect his fear and think less of him. He had less problem with strangers whom he might never meet again, but still felt a disgust for himself each time he was compelled to avoid public toilet urination for whatever reason. By the time he consulted us, he had become obsessed and depressed by his phobia. He stated that, if he didn't overcome the problem, it might eventually hamper his career development. Treatment involved: (1) imaginal flooding, (2) *in vivo* flooding with therapist, (3) cognitive restructuring, and (4) homework.

For public urination fear, imaginal flooding serves as a rehearsal for the *in vivo* flooding. Since some of Mr. J.'s fear resulted in a concern about his future career, we also had him imagine implosive scenes where co-workers actually ridiculed him for his fear. These scenes involved the usual aggression, counter-aggression, and punishment themes commonly used in implosive therapy. *In vivo* flooding was carried out in the public restroom at the therapist's office building. The client was asked to come to the session with a full bladder. On arrival, he was required to stand at the urinal for as long as it took for him to relax his bladder and urinate. If he could not urinate within 20 minutes, he was allowed to leave the restroom or to use the stall. Regardless of success, Mr. J. was required to continue standing at the urinal for at least three minutes after he urinated. This procedure was used on the theory that standing at the urinal under relatively lower anxiety conditions might bring about more neutral stimulus associations to the client's urinal standing behavior. On the third session, Mr. J. successfully voided in the urinal for the first time. Cognitive restructuring and thought-stopping using paradoxical intention were taught to help Mr. J. interrupt anxiety-provoking thoughts while standing at the urinal. For example, instead of his usual thought that someone might come in and find out about his fear, he was instructed to say to himself, "I hope someone does come in, I don't care about them, and it will give me an opportunity to stand here and extinguish this silly fear."

Homework involved instructions to the client to practice his *in vivo* assignment. It was necessary to grade this exposure, starting with relatively safe toilets, such as urinating in a stall with a commode but leaving the door unlocked, and working up to more anxiety-provoking restrooms like those at his work.

Mr. J. made rapid progress and felt he could handle his fear after four sessions and four weeks of homework; but even at one year follow-up, Mr. J. reported that he still might have problems at work if he tried to void in the urinal with anything less than a full bladder.

Agoraphobia

The term *agoraphobia* is derived from the Greek word *agora* meaning marketplace or public place, and, of course, *phobia* or fear. The psychiatric disorder of agoraphobia involves a generalized fear of leaving a place of safety, such as one's home or spouse. When not in a "safe place," agoraphobics fear that they may become trapped and lose control of themselves. Many have panic attacks. Those that do fear a panic attack usually anticipate one of several disasterous results such as (1) fainting, (2) "going crazy," (3) uncontrolled striking out, and/or worst of all (4) dying. The fear is usually experienced in crowded places where the patient cannot readily escape to safety. The middle of a crowded shopping center, an airplane, or a car are common examples of places where agoraphobics fear they will become "trapped," and be unable to escape and reach help. The more accessible the agoraphobic is to "help," the less anxiety is experienced. Help is usually defined as returning to a safe place where a close friend or relative is waiting. Thus, most agoraphobics remain acutely aware of just how far they are from home or from a significant other, or where doctors' offices and hospitals are located. More importantly perhaps is that they are constantly assessing how difficult it might be for them to extricate themselves from an "unsafe" situation.

The severe panic reactions experienced by many agoraphobics include symptoms of hyperventilation, rapid heart rate, dizziness, and fainting. The sufferer is greatly sensitive to his or her potential to panic and therefore may have a tendency to interpret normal internal sensations are signaling an impending attack. For example, climbing a flight of stairs may precipitate a panic attack because the physical exertion increases heart rate and felt heart beat force. The agoraphobic may then construe these normal palpitations as dangerous, thereby bringing about a full-blown panic attack.

For agoraphobics the feeling of "trappedness" is central to their discomfort. The most dangerous traps are where people demand attention, where interaction is required with others, and where one cannot innocuously escape. A common example of a dangerous place for agoraphobics is standing in the middle of a grocery line waiting to be checked out at the counter. Moreover, many agoraphobics also fear that they will some day experience a panic attack that will never abate and that, consequently, they will therefore remain in a constant state of extreme fear. In a literal sense, the most basic fear for the agoraphobic is fear itself.

Agoraphobia is more common among women then men. Women who suffer from this disorder often feel housebound or that they can only venture short distances from their home. In addition, most married agoraphobics are only able to leave home when accompanied by a spouse or child. The onset of symptoms for both sexes is generally between the ages of 15 and 35.

For most agoraphobics, we begin individual therapy with imaginal flooding or implosive therapy, which is then followed by *in vivo* flooding and homework. The initial imaginal flooding accomplishes three objectives: (1) it serves as a rehearsal to better prepare patients to properly carry out the *in vivo* procedure; (2) it reduces anxiety about the *in vivo* treatment procedure to come, and (3) it directly reduces anxiety associated with the stimulus cue.

As reported in Chapter 3, session length appears to be another important factor. Long *in vivo* exposure sessions of up to three hours are more effective than short sessions, even if the total treatment time is held constant. Yet, long sessions are often impractical for many therapists. It is best to keep in mind that regardless of session length, the most important component to any treatment program for agoraphobics is multiple, repeated exposure to the feared situation. Patients are asked to look for opportunities to expose themselves to feared situations and to take advantage of these opportunities as much as possible. Also, agoraphobics respond well to group treatment. For reasons already given, however, only individual treatment will be discussed in this chapter. For those therapists who are interested in using a group approach, we recommend the method proposed by Chambless and Goldstein (1981).

Finally, unlike simple phobics, most agoraphobics have severe personality problems that interact with their fears. For example, we agree with Chambless and Goldstein (1981), who present evidence that "certain person variables interact with prolonged stress to lead to agoraphobia." These person variables include (1) a hysterical cognitive style, (2) lack of assertion, (3) a sense of low self-sufficiency, due either to lack of skills or separation sensitivity; and (4) a predisposition to panic attacks. Under such conditions Chambless and Goldstein theorize that fear develops from three sources: (1) conditioned anxiety to interoceptive cues or tension, (2) second-order conditioning of places, and (3) catastrophic cognitions about "loss of control." Thus flooding alone is unsuccessful for some agoraphobics. We find that clients who evidence these personality problems are more likely to stay in therapy if these person variables receive therapeutic attention.

Case Study

Mrs. B., a 46-year-old white female, was a typical agoraphobic. She had been married for 20 years and had two children, a boy 16 living at home and a recently married daughter. She was a nonassertive person who had never worked outside the home. Her fears had no obvious point of onset, but had gradually worsened over the years. Her husband was tolerant and supportive. He rarely complained about his wife's behavior and never made demands on her to change, even though her fears made life inconvenient for him. He did the shopping and ran most of the errands. Social life was almost nonexistant, except for an occasional dinner for invited guests. Reciprocal invitations however were always turned down. This resulted in embarrassment for both parties.

The patient had never sought treatment before. She stated that she had not considered her problem treatable and was unaware that medical or psychiatric help was an option. She consulted one of us after reading about our treatment program in a local newpaper. Her therapy goals were to be able to drive a car alone and to go to the grocery store and shopping centers by herself without anxiety.

Symptoms were typical. If she were in a large grocery store or in a shopping center and was not close to an exit, she would begin to panic. The feeling was described as one of an overpowering fear that she would faint, fall on the floor, or otherwise make a spectacle of herself. The feeling was described as a typical anxiety or panic attack and included the sensations of light headedness, a feeling that her vision was blurring and becoming tunnel-like, and that her surroundings were closing in on her. Her pulse would quicken, her chest would tighten and, at its worst, these sensations were described as a fear that she was dying or that something terrible was about to happen. She realized that all of this was irrational and stated that she knew she was in perfect health. During the attacks, these feelings were so intense and overpowering that it was impossible for her to control of calm herself. Like many other agoraphobics, Mrs. B. reported that she had never actually lost consciousness during any of the panic episodes. Perhaps more important than the panic attack itself was her feeling of being trapped. She noted, as do many agoraphobics, that the panic attacks were uncomfortable but they were made much worse by the fact that she felt she could not remove herself from the situation and that others would observe her in panic.

During early sessions Mrs. B. was asked to imagine herself inside a shopping center without access to a door. She was encouraged to experience the panic as much as possible, but was not asked to imagine anything other than the feelings and situations she had already experienced (flooding). (In contrast, in implosive therapy the client might be encouraged to imagine passing out and then waking up with many people standing around and staring at her.)

Next Mrs. B. was accompanied by one of us and her husband to a local shopping area. The primary purpose of the trip was to instruct both patient and spouse in the *in vivo* flooding procedure. In the past, Mrs. B. had always avoided being alone in a shopping area. She was instructed to go into the store alone, to remain just inside the door for a time, and then return to the therapist. She was asked to repeat the exercise until she felt comfortable. Next, she was asked to go further into the store, remain for several minutes and to return again, repeating this until she felt comfortable. Flooding patients are encouraged not to be concerned about their anxiety level unless they feel a "full-blown anxiety attack coming on." Successful completion of each trial is rewarded by constant reassurance.

Patients are taught to realize that if they remain in the dangerous situation long enough, anxiety levels will eventually abate. Most important, clients are instructed never to leave the frightening situation while they are in a panic or while they feel very uncomfortable. They are told to wait until the anxiety subsides. This, of course, is a departure from past experience. This procedure reduces the likelihood of reinforcing the avoidance response through fear reduction.

After being instructed in the above procedure, Mrs. B. was encouraged to continue *in vivo* therapy on her own at home. Therapy contracts defined the amount of time she agreed to stay in the "dangerous" environment each day. She was also asked to keep a diary of when she went out and how she felt both before, during, and after her homework assignment. This client met with the therapist two times per week for the first 4 weeks and then once per week thereafter. The number and timing of therapy sessions will, of course, depend on the individual patient. It is best to see patients at least twice per week initially. Intensive treatment increases the likelihood that clients will stay in therapy. Agoraphobics tend to cancel sessions and discontinue therapy at a higher rate than do most other types of psychotherapy patients. This can be avoided by having clients pay in advance and by demonstrating to them early in therapy that the technique is successful. At each therapy session new therapy contracts were determined. In the above case, homework sessions were the most practical method of exposing this client to the feared environment. This was possible because the client's spouse was willing to help. If such support is not available, more active therapist participation in the *in vivo* flooding aspect of the treatment will be necessary. As noted previously, there is data to suggest that for agoraphobics, homework alone can be as effective as having the therapist actually involved in the *in vivo* treatment (Griest, Marks, Berlin, Gournay, & Noshirvani, 1980; Mathews *et al.*, 1977). The use of homework in contracting for goals on a session-by-session basis, also has the advantage of allowing patients to experience success in the environment that is of more direct concern to them. This reduces the chances that any extinction or habituation occurring under therapist directed *in vivo* exposure would not generalize to the specific environment of concern to the patient. The disadvantage, of course, is that the therapist has less control over the treatment process . Also spouses or significant others often inadvertently reinforce phobic behavior. In this case, for example, in an effort to help his wife remain comfortable, the spouse had discouraged the client from trying to function autonomously. The therapist must be observant and careful with instructions to spouses. Even though it may appear inconvenient to live with an agoraphobic, it can have its advantages. A jealous spouse doesn't have to worry about his partner having affairs with others. Furthermore, female agoraphobics are usually excellent housekeepers and mothers. If the significant other does find the client's dependence rewarding, any progress toward independent functioning will threaten that relationship and must be considered in therapy. We suggest that the therapist deal with this issue in individual sessions with the significant other and with follow-up joint sessions, if necessary.

As noted, Mrs. B. complained of panic attacks. If the panic attack interferes with exposure (i.e., the client is unable to adequately perceive the environment) it may be helpful to train clients in panic control. Several self-control techniques are effective in helping to control panic attacks. Patients are instructed that if they feel an attack coming on they should: (1) look down to the floor or ground, (2) find a place to sit down, (3) take two, slow, even deep breaths, extending the stomach and lower diaphragm, (4) close their eyes and refocus their attention by remembering the therapist's reassurance that they will not die or faint, and (5) systematically start to relax various muscle groups starting with the head and shoulders. For patients who have problems relaxing, a formal relaxation program such as progressive muscle relaxation can be offered. Simple meditation exercises can also be helpful in abating panic attacks. Another technique that helps control oncoming panic is to have clients wear a rubber band around the wrist with instructions to "snap it hard" when they start to feel the panic symptoms. This procedure has been successful for obsessional-thought problems, but is also efficacious any time attention refocusing is desired. In the above example, the client did not feel that she would be able to use the rubber band effectively, but did use and was helped by the other panic control techniques. Weeks (1970) has offered several cognitive techniques to help control panic. She advises patients to "float" or "go" with the panic, not to fight it, and to let it run its course. This, she feels, will prevent patients from developing a secondary fear of fear that increases the panic feeling. This ploy seems consistent with exposure technique. We must again emphasize that after the panic abates to encourage the client to return to or stay in the feared situation and never leave it while in panic.

Rational therapy for agoraphobics without exposure is probably ineffective. In Mrs. B's case, however, we encouraged her to consider her fears from a rational viewpoint in order to refocus attention. She was strongly encouraged to be acutely aware of the irrationality of her behavior in the "dangerous environment." Most clients will complain that they already know it is irrational, but have difficulty being rational during periods of high anxiety. Thoughts of dread and doom overpower any rational analysis. Nevertheless, we have found that if clients practice rational thinking about their symptoms, they will eventually learn to prevent panic through rational self-talk.

Finally, follow-up is very important in treating agoraphobia. Almost all patients, especially extremely nonassertive clients such as Mrs. B. will lose some of their gains if they are not strongly encouraged to continue to fight against their inclination to avoid the feared situation. Agoraphobics are avoiders, and their tendency to remove themselves from uncomfortable situations for the immediate reward of anxiety reduction is strong since this behavior has been practiced and reinforced over many years.

Mrs. B. was moderately successful in attaining her goals, but was still not completely comfortable driving alone at one year following 15 individual therapy sessions and many hours of homework. She did do the shopping for the family and reported that she was still working on her fears.

CASE STUDY

Mrs. C., a 35-year-old married female suffering from agoraphobia, presented with numerous fears, including those of being alone, of driving, of elevators, and of flying. Mrs. C. described a traumatic home life in which she felt trapped between angry parents and unable to express her own anger for fear of desertion. Her first anxiety attack occurred when she was 15 years old and driving about 30 miles away from home with both of her parents. Her hands shook, her knees were weak, she felt dizzy, had stomach pains with diarrhea, hyperventilated, broke into a cold sweat, and feared she was going crazy. Soon after that, a girlfriend in her class did "go crazy" and was "locked-up" three times that year. The patient also read a novel (*The Snake Pit*) presenting a stereotyped view of a restrictive mental hospital. That same year she had her appendix removed and afterwards had anxiety and depressive attacks everyday at lunch. She would sit between her mother and father who would argue and bait each other. Afterwards, she would go to her room and cry for hours while shaking and having diarrhea. Her parents ignored this behavior and she gradually became very angry at them for not taking her to a doctor.

She described her father as extremely cold and unloving. He was constantly physically ill and she had to wait on him hand and foot. Her mother was described as anxious, rigid, paranoid, and accusatory. She, like the patient, was evidently extremely angry at the "sick" father. The patient attempted to be their therapist in order to keep them together and prevent them from deserting her, all the while feeling trapped and hating them both. The patient's fear of flying dated back to an incident when her mother asked her to fly home because her dad was "dying." She went, even though she was angry at herself for going and at her parents for asking her. She had been called home two to three times per year for the past 15 years because her father was reported to be on the verge of death. On each occasion, she ended up sitting in her father's hospital room, and observing her parents fight and accuse each other. The particular incident that initiated the flying fear was long and involved and, as is frequently done, the patient was asked to write out the incident in detail. Her report of the incident ran to 7 type-written pages. In brief, on her return flight, she was feeling extremely frustrated and angry toward her parents and her husband, as well as guilty for wishing that her father would die. She was feeling trapped in these various relationships, as well as on the plane, and a severe anxiety attack ensued and henceforth she was afraid to fly.

Mrs. C. had a very strong fear of abandonment. When she was three years old, she vividly recalled being lost in a corn field and being able to hear her parents calling but unable to find them. She felt very panicked. A few years later, her parents went on vacation and she recalls her grandmother telling her that her parents did not love her and were never coming back. Apparently, due to these fears of abandonment, she reported getting very anxious when she felt angry and when her husband was angry at her. Pushed for what would be the worst thing that could happen to her, she stated that if both her husband and her mother died or otherwise left her, she feared that this would lead to her going crazy. She would then end up in a mental hospital where she would be trapped. Because many of Mrs. C.'s fears were imaginal and hypothetical, treatment entailed implosive scenes followed by *in vivo* exposure.

In the third therapy session, the first implosive scene was presented and it dealt with her fears of abandonment. In this scene, she was three years old and lost in a corn field. She was alone, cold, hungry, and frightened. All her needs for caring, nourishment, and touch were unmet. And in fact, her parents didn't care for her, indeed they hated her and wished she had never been born. This scene of being lost, alone, and rejected by her primary care givers was drawn out extensively. Eventually, in the scene she died and was buried in a small, tight coffin, and again cues were presented suggesting that no one cared and that they were glad she was dead. Mrs. C. gave this scene a discomfort rating of 50 and reported that she was aware of holding herself back and of being afraid to let herself really feel alone, abandoned, and trapped. The scene was assigned as homework. In the fourth session, she reported having performed the homework scene 10 times with anxiety decreasing from a rating of 50 to 15. However, she continued to prevent herself from totally experiencing the feeling of desertion.

In the fifth session, an implosive scene was presented in which she was pictured as a 15-year old at the dinner table with her mother "bitching" at her father and, to a lesser extent, at her. The client observed and experienced this in some detail, feeling increasingly angry and sick to her stomach and trapped in the situation, until she finally exploded, told her mother off repeatedly, and finally beat and kicked her mother to death. The client had difficulty imagining hitting her mother but appeared extremely angry and tense during the scene and afterwards gave it an anger rating of 95. The scene was assigned as homework. In the following session, Mrs. C. reported that she had performed the scene once a day with anger decreasing from a rating of 90 to 70. She also reported that, while performing the homework scene, she became aware of some anger directed at her father. A scene was presented in which Mrs. C. was pictured feeling very angry at her father because he ordered her mother to pick some strawberries which made her mother cry. Her father responded "Your crying is making me sick." In the scene, her father was pictured as telling the patient to get down and help her mother. But the client stubbornly refused saying, "You are not going to walk on me." The father was then pictured as actually walking on the client, hitting her and kicking her until she finally angrily told him off, kicked him and beat him. During the scene, she expressed a great deal of anger, but afterwards felt relaxed and triumphant saying she wished she had been able to express anger overtly at her father in her younger days. This scene was assigned as homework. Two weeks later, the client had accomplished the homework scene 18 times with the emotional rating declining from 80 to 30.

The implosive scene presented in the sixth session essentially recreated the first time she had an anxiety attack on an airplane, (when she was flying home from her visit with her "dying" father). Anxiety was rated at 85. In the following session, the patient reported attempting this scene once per day but she experienced relatively low anxiety due to various avoidance maneuvers. The scene was repeated in the session with the patient again being pictured trapped on the plane, unable to avoid it in any way. This resulted in an anxiety rating of 95 and the scene was again assigned as homework.

In the eighth session, she reported performing the homework scene one to two times per day with anxiety decreasing from 80 to 40. She reported that in two weeks she had a chance to go on a vacation but that it would involve taking a car ferry for about 30 minutes. As with cars and planes, she very much feared being trapped in the boat in the middle of the water and experiencing an anxiety attack. Consequently, a scene was presented that pictured just that happening—being on the ferry, getting very anxious, having an anxiety attack, losing control and going crazy. The scene was assigned as homework.

The next session again repeated this same scene with the same homework assignment and, one week later, she was able to take the ferry on her vacation.

The next three sessions involved *in vivo* exposure to flying in an airplane, riding in an elevator, and traveling in a car with someone else and by herself. Following treatment, Mrs. C. was able to take all these means of conveyance without feeling trapped or anxious, and was also able to visit her mother without feeling trapped or inappropriately angry or anxious. These changes were maintained at 6 months, though she reported fearing lengthy commercial plane rides. She had nonetheless engaged in such rides without incidence.

Panic Disorders

Panic attacks may occur as part of several of the various anxiety disorders. As already noted, agoraphobics often experience panic attacks. In fact, DSM-III distinguishes between agoraphobia with and without panic attacks. Sometimes panic appears to be the client's only symptom. In these cases, the client does not limit his or her activity but experiences panic apparently unrelated to any stimulus event. Many symptoms are common during panic: dyspnea, palpitations, chest pain or discomfort, choking or smothering sensations, dizziness, vertigo, unsteady feelings, feelings of unreality, paresthesias, hot and cold flashes, sweating, faintness, and trembling or shaking. As noted above, treatment for panic is accomplished by having the client counteract the symptoms with a combination of relaxation and cognitive restructuring. Depending on the particular situation, clients are usually trained in some form of relaxation and are instructed to use relaxation exercises at the first sign of panic. Slow deep breathing exercises may be helpful. Where hyperventilation is severe, relief may be obtained by breath holding or by rebreathing into a paper bag (this may require a minute or more for symptom relief). We also ask some clients to wear a rubber band around their wrist, and snap it hard when they feel they are about to experience a full-blown panic attack. Cognitive restructuring can be accomplished by having the client remember the therapist's reassurance that there is no real danger and to combat the catastrophic fantasies, such as thoughts of death or insanity, by focusing on a predetermined pleasant fantasy or memory.

Treatment of panic can be accompanied by the use of implosive scenes that expose the clients to their particular catastrophic fantasies. Such fantasies include fears of going insane, losing control, and death. The following scene is an example if a typical implosive theme that might be used with a client who feared that he would go insane.

CASE STUDY

Gerald, a 31-year-old laborer, was treated as an inpatient. He feared his anxiety would become so great that he would lose control of himself, go insane, and ultimately die. The implosive scene used to extinguish this fear is transcribed below.

T. Make this as real as possible. Let's begin by supposing that our session has actually ended and you are on your way out of my office and walking back toward your room, a very familiar path. You have walked this way many times before. You can walk and look about you, catch glimpses of the hallway, floors, nurses, and aides walking about as well as other patients. You are feeling happy because this is the day you are going to leave the hospital and you are feeling that this hospitalization has been one of your best: you've been at your best. You haven't had a serious problem as you usually do. But then, all of a sudden Dr. Smith walks up to you. Try to look at his face. He tips his head to the side, the way he usually does when he is going to make a pronouncement of some kind, and you begin to wonder what is on his mind. What's he going to say? Maybe he is going to tell you that you are okay and to go down and pick up your clothes to leave the hospital. But instead, he looks at you and says, "Gerald, I am very sorry to have to tell you this, but Dr. Jones and I, in going over records of your past hospitalizations, have decided that we can't release you at the present time. You have to understand that this is nothing against you, but we have a legal responsibility in this case. We feel that you are dangerous to yourself." Try to experience the kind of anxiety, anger, depression, and sadness which you feel if he had actually said this to you. Try to feel that anxiety as he tells you that you are dangerous to yourself and others. They have decided that they have to call you a hopeless, paranoid schizophrenic. There is no telling at what point you might turn into a killer or a suicidal person! This is what he says to you and that therefore they have instituted commitment proceedings against you and that, without telling you, they have obtained by the use of two psychiatrists and your wife, commitment papers. Try to feel the anxiety. Don't fight it—try to feel as much as you can. That's good. The more anxious you get, the more you should try to feel the anxiety. They have decided to commit you.Think about the idea of commitment as intensely as you can. Don't put it out of your mind. Keep it right in the center of your mind. These three people have committed you. And Dr. Smith further informs you that, rather than staying here, since this is not a long-term hospital and your treatment will undoubtedly be long-term, you will have to be sent to another hospital. Now try to see yourself as you would be—anxious, upset, and you don't really believe that you are dangerous. Yet, on the other hand, the doctors had told you so. How are you feeling right now? What can you do? What can you add to this scene? Tell me how you are feeling.

C. Sad.

T. OK. What can you see? What are you experiencing at this moment?

C. *(Sighing)* These are the thoughts I have had.

T. Can you add anything to it?

C. I can't live locked-up.

T. Right. That's no kind of life for a human being. This is the thought that goes through your head.

C. *(Breathes heavily)*

T. They are treating you like some kind of dangerous animal; like a mad dog, not like a human being. You feel sad, but you also feel angry. You feel frustrated. You feel afraid. You don't know what's waiting for you in the long-term hospital because they lied to you once. They have told you that you were going to leave and now they are committing you instead. Now try to see yourself being sent in the car to the hospital. You are not aware of much of the drive up there. You are being transferred with several other patients. Your belongings are in the trunk of the car. Because you are so shocked and stunned about the whole thing you hardly know how you got there. But soon you see yourself arriving. You see this hospital stuck out in the middle of no where, a bunch of old buildings, a God-forsaken place. When you are admitted to the hospital, you begin to see all kinds of chronic patients shuffling on the wards. Some of them look like they may have been lobotomized; some of them look like they may have had dozens and dozens of shock treatments. They can't even remember where they are anymore. And when you get to this hospital and you get settled in your room, you have to go before a staff conference and you can see the people sitting around. You're expected to sit in a chair and be interviewed by them. You know you have to make a good impression on them but you are so anxious you find it very difficult to do so. You have got to convince them that you shouldn't be committed. Maybe these people will listen to you. You begin to develop some hope again. Maybe there is somebody here who can be trusted. Maybe there is somebody here who will listen to you and understand that you are not the kind of person that others said you were. Try to picture the people sitting around the table and yourself, just as you would be at a job interview or any other interview, the center of attention. They are looking at you . They are watching your every move, to see if there is anything they can determine that would confirm the judgment made about you that you were paranoid schizophrenic; that you deserved to be committed for protection of society and they begin asking you some questions. And one doctor down at the end of the table, who looks very much like Dr. Smith, asks you a very odd question. He says something like, "Well, what about those radio receiving units that were in your shoes anyway?" You don't know what to do. It sounds like an odd question. How could he possibly know about that. Are you seeing this? Is this real? And yet if he really is there and you don't answer, they are going to think that is odd, too. So you are asking him to repeat the question and everybody stares at you because there really wasn't anyone there, and you are talking to an empty chair and they think they know that you are really as psychotic as everyone has said you are. And again with the same long face they say, "Well, we are very sorry about this Gerald but this is for your own good. You are going to have to have a series of electric shock treatments. Do you know what this is a polite term for? Have you seen people who have had these kinds of treatments?" At this point, try to imagine yourself becoming frightened. Try to imagine yourself beginning to lose control completely, screaming that you don't want these treatments. You are a big person so you are able to fight them off for a while but they get four or five aides around you. You are trying to throw them off. You are trying to fight them off because you don't want to have your head ruined by these treatments. You don't want to be turned into a vegetable. But they are going to do it. They grab you and they drag you towards the room where you can see the shock machine, the dials, the switches sitting on the table. You can see the electrodes on the paddles that are put on the sides of the person's head. You can see the nurse waiting for you and the whole place smells like medicine, like anesthetic. They throw you up on the table and they strap your arms down. Try to imagine yourself struggling and there is nothing you can do. You are completely helpless. They apply the current and then you see an arch of light go past your eyes and you lose consciousness.

Obsessive-Compulsive Disorders

Obsessions are defined as either thoughts or images that are egodystonic or not experienced as being produced internally. People who suffer from severe obsessions experience the thoughts as intrusive, or somehow being forced into their mind. They feel powerless to rid themselves of the thoughts. Most feel that they need to resist the thoughts and, when they are unable to extricate them, anxiety is generated. Obsessional thoughts are often experienced as senseless and aversive. Obsessions usually involve fear of causing harm to oneself or others, loss of control, pervasive doubts, and sexual and religious fears (Foa & Steketee, 1979).

Compulsions refer to behavior. The intent of these behaviors is usually to reduce the anxiety caused by obsessions or to "control" obsessions. Foa and Steketee (1979), in an excellent review of the symptoms and treatments of obsessive-compulsive disorders, point out that obsessions may be seen as a type of phobic stimulus, and the compulsive behavior as the avoidance response aimed at reducing the anxiety associated with this stimulus.

Most patients who suffer from this disorder experience both the intrusive thoughts and compulsive rituals. However, some only experience the thoughts or images while other individuals carry out senseless rituals without obsessional thoughts, but these are seldom considered pathological.

Most obsessive-compulsive disorders involve two types of compulsions, called "washers" and "checkers." Washers feel contaminated, usually when they touch or are in the presence of specified objects, people, or situations. Constant washing is necessary to rid themselves of the contamination. Washers usually realize that they are not actually contaminated by germs or dirt but feel contaminated in a more abstract manner. Washing a contaminated part of the body is often carried out in a ritualistic manner similar to a surgeon scrubbing.

Checkers suffer from the strong urge to repeatedly assure themselves that they have or can carry out a specified activity. Often this will involve checking specific, potentially dangerous appliances several times to ascertain that they have been turned off. Another common type of checker is one who feels the constant urge to check doors and windows to make sure they are locked. Often checkers have ritualized their checking behavior such that they cannot feel comfortable until they have checked and rechecked the object a specified number of times.

Individuals who suffer from obsessive-compulsive disorders are usually above average in intelligence. The disorder is chronic, with symptoms becoming more severe during stressful periods in the individual's life. Depression often accompanies exacerbation of the obsessive-compulsive symptoms and is often a factor in treatment. Onset is usually in late adolescence or early adulthood, but in some cases begins in childhood.

As already noted, flooding or, more precisely, response prevention is an effective treatment for obsessive-compulsive disorder. Response prevention requires that clients force themselves not to behave compulsively and simply to experience the anxiety until it habituates on its own. Most clients resist such treatment at first on the grounds that they "can't stand it" and require that the therapist take a relatively more graded approach. Often we start with clients by agreeing to allow them to hold off the performance of the ritual for a specified period of time (e.g., if they have the urge to check something a second time, they are asked to hold off checking it for an hour). As treatment progresses, they are required to increase the time between urge and checking. Often a combination of *in vivo* flooding and response prevention is effective. For example, one of our clients who had a number of compulsions would check 50–60 times to see whether a door was locked before she could sleep. She also had rituals that required her to take her clothes off in a special manner, sometimes taking up to an hour just to hang up one dress. Obsessional fears included concerns that she might drop and break things in a manner that would allow pieces of the broken object to fly up and cut her face. Thus, she could not wash dishes. Treatment involved both response prevention for checking behavior and more active flooding of the obsessions. For dress hanging behavior, the patient was required to take all her clothes off the hangers and rehang each one "improperly." She was instructed to break a dish on purpose on the floor and to leave the pieces on the floor for at least an hour. In therapy, compulsives should be rewarded for not giving into the urges. We tell them to "push against" the urges as much as possible. Another flooding procedure that is helpful with obsessive-compulsive clients is to use response prevention for compulsive rituals or behaviors that do not bother the client. These might include minor compulsions such as mildly excessive neatness in dress or in manner. Flooding might involve having the client be purposely slovenly or practice not completing certain simple tasks.

In most cases, *in vivo* treatment of compulsive behaviors through response prevention is enough to allow exposure to the obsessions. We find, however, that specific imaginal scenes directed at having the client practice the obsessional thoughts in imagination, even when they do not feel compelled to do so, can be helpful. This often goes beyond simply flooding the obsessions. Many clients who experience guilt or anxiety over obsessional thoughts tend to avoid thinking about the consequences of their actions. Thus, for example, if a patient has a guilt-producing hostile thought about a friend in which he or she imagines hurting that person, we also encourage the client to practice imagining what might happen if he or she were to carry out the behavior. These scenes usually involve punishment and/or counteraggression and sometimes tap significant unconscious fears. In imaginal flooding of obsessions, a good rule is that it is better to overexpose rather than underexpose.

In most cases, compulsive behaviors offer at least temporary relief from anxiety. In many severe cases, however, the compulsive behaviors themselves cause guilt. The following case demonstrates this problem. The primary techniques used were implosive therapy, flooding in imagination, and response prevention. The case also demonstrates the difference between flooding and negative practice. Negative practice is often confused with flooding when working with severe obsessive-compulsive disorders. In this case, the therapist who treated this client prior to her referral to us used a form of negative practice that may have exacerbated her symptoms.

Case Study

Marsha was a 28-year-old white housewife and interior decorator. During the year prior to her referral, she had suffered from obsessions and compulsions, had been seen by two other psychotherapists, and had been hospitalized twice for severe depression and suicidal ideation. She was referred by her therapist, an analyst, for "behavioral treatment of her symptoms." The analyst was not using psychoanalysis with her but was seeing her primarily for support and to adjust her antidepressant medications. He continued to see her throughout most of the treatment. Treatment was carried out in 22 sessions over a five month period.

Marsha's primary complaint was that, since the birth of her first and only daughter (approximately one year prior to her referral), she had experienced "visual thoughts" that would uncontrollably come into her mind. The thoughts centered on the fear that she might harm her daughter in some manner. These obsessive thoughts took a variety of forms, including sticking sharp objects, such as scissors or a knife, in the child's eye, throwing boiling water on her, putting her in the fireplace, throwing hot grease on her, or driving over her with the car. These were only a few of the more than 30 types of aggressive-obsessional experiences that Marsha engaged in before and during treatment. She complained that the thoughts entered her mind "in a flash" against her will and that she seemed incapable of dismissing them until they had run their course. Her concern was that she might actually act out the thoughts, even though she did not want to do so. She felt that, because she could not control her thoughts, she might also at some point lose control and actually carry out the behaviors. The thoughts produced considerable anxiety and also increased her guilt. Marsha felt that if she had these thoughts, even though she consciously did not want them, she must at some level of consciousness wish to harm her daughter.

The compulsive behaviors that brought some short-term relief from the thoughts were essentially checking behaviors with Marsha "checking out" her control by starting to carry out the aggressive act but not following through. Compulsive behaviors included holding a skillet of hot bacon grease near the child's face and then pulling the pan away, holding the child near the fireplace and then pulling her away and, while the child slept, holding a pair of scissors close to the child's eyes for a few seconds and then pulling them away. When she realized that she had control and couldn't carry out the act, she was relieved for a few minutes to a few hours. However, as the obsessions continued, the compulsive maneuvers became less effective in reducing anxiety. When she first started having the obsession, engaging in the compulsive behavior would relieve the anxiety for several days. By the time she was referred to us, her relief would last only a few minutes. Her guilt resulted from thinking "what if" she had slipped or "what if" the child had awakened and had pulled her head up into the sharp object.

Although Marsha carried out these acts thousands of times during the child's first two years of life, she never harmed the child in any way. On the contrary, one of Marsha's problems stemming from her compulsive behavior was that she was so guilty over her behavior that she could not effectively set limits for the child.

By the time Marsha was referred, several other factors exacerbated her problem. Since she did not trust herself to be alone with the child when her husband was at work, she would spend most of her time at her mother's house. She was also experiencing both vegetative and psychological symptoms of depression that would leave her enervated and unable to maintain the household, as well as uninterested and unmotivated in maintaining a touching relationship with her husband. These factors, along with the financial burden of the hospitalization and therapy, had put a severe strain on her marital relationship. Marsha feared that, if she did not get control of her thoughts and behaviors, her husband would be forced, out of fear for the safety of their child, to separate from her and take the child. In reality, however, her husband was not overly concerned that she would harm the child and, as far as is known, never considered such a separation at any time during treatment.

Marsha's past history was fairly unremarkable but significant. She was born and raised near where she presently lived. Her family consisted of two older brothers, her mother and father, all of whom still lived in the same small, urban community. She described her mother as overprotective and traditional, and her father was seen as strong and controlling. She described herself as a "model child" and rarely a discipline problem. She received above average grades in school, graduated from high school and received an Associate Arts Degree in merchandising. She married at age 21. Although she was raised in a religious family, she only occasionally attended church as an adult and at the time of treatment was considering converting from the Baptist denomination to Catholicism, her husband's religion.

One of Marsha's most significant early memories occurred at the age of nine when she attended the funeral of a family friend's three-year-old. The child had died as a result of burns received from pulling a pot of hot grease off the stove, and spilling it over her head and body. Marsha also recalled that her mother had often cautioned her to be careful in the kitchen. Her mother's constant message was that the world was a dangerous place and that, if you were not careful, you could easily get hurt.

Marsha had seen two therapists prior to being referred. The first one suggested a negative practice technique. Marsha was instructed to engage purposely in the various compulsive behaviors without any imaginal flooding. This tactic had no positive effect and, according to Marsha, only made matters worse, making her feel even more guilty with little anxiety relief. Negative practice is not the same as flooding. Marsha's compulsive behavior was not, in itself, fear-producing but rather fear avoiding. In effect, what the therapist was doing was having her engage in the avoidance behavior. There is no evidence that negative practice is effective with compulsive behavior (Boudewyns & Shipley, 1982). We suggested that Marsha make every effort not to engage in the behaviors. In general, when treating obsessive-compulsive patients, effective therapy will almost always include this type of *response prevention* that, in effect, exposes the client to the fear produced by the obsessional thoughts.

The etiology of the obsession was significant. When Marsha's child was born, she initially had many fears for her safety. She recalled her mother's reminders of how vulnerable children were and how they must constantly be protected from their environment. Everytime the baby would cry, Marsha's immediate thought was that something awful might be happening. She began to feel guilty anytime she was not directly attending the child. As she felt more tied down by the baby, she also became more frustrated and more easily angered by the child's demands. The anger motivated her to avoid the baby, but avoidance only made her feel guilty and increased her fears (and images) that the child would be harmed. It was hypothesized that Marsha often had visual images of the baby having an accident, while at the same time feeling angry at the child for demanding so much. This association led Marsha to interpret her obsessional images as "wishes" and to visualize herself as the perpetrator of the accidents. At this point, she doubted her own motives and began to "check" her ability to harm the child with the compulsive behaviors. Thus began for Marsha the constant vacillation between guilt and anxiety.

Treatment consisted of thought stopping, response prevention, procedures to control irrational thinking, and implosive therapy. To help control the behaviors, Marsha wore a rubber band on her wrist and snapped it when the urge to behave compulsively became strong. We also suggested alternative behaviors that would inhibit the compulsive response such as leaving the house, reading, turning on the television, etc. She was asked to remind herself constantly that it was OK to *think* harm to her child, and she was given the rationale that everyone feels this way at times. She was encouraged to repeatedly and purposely visualize scenes of harming the baby until it didn't bother her. One typical scene is transcribed below.

T. Close your eyes. OK, now. Maybe we can go through a scene with Karen. Let's try to imagine yourself actually doing it. I want you to start thinking about taking a sharp object, putting it to her face. You walk in and see her face. You take the pencil and you put it up to her. You feel yourself getting more and more overwhelmed by the urge and you are holding back just as if somebody is almost forcing your arms to move. Can you see her now as you do this?
C. Uh-huh.
T. Feel it now. You are looking at her and you see her eyes and your pencil. You start to push it in. Feel the urge become greater and greater. And you start to feel that sinking feeling like it is slipping away. It is like you can't control your hands now.
C. Uh.
T. You lose control of your hands. Something snaps in your mind. It is like you are not yourself and you see that pencil there and you see Karen, you don't want to do it, but you watch your hand with the pencil start moving closer and closer to her. See that? See her there looking up at you?
C. Uh-huh.
T. The pencil is getting closer and closer to her and then something snaps and you lose control. You can't help it and your hands say, "Take that pencil and push it into her face." Can you see that?
C. Uh-huh.
T. Back it up and see it again. It is important to try to see it. Not just before and the aftermath, but actually doing it.
C. I just can't. *(Crying)*
T. Take the pencil now. Go ahead. You have got the pencil in your hand. Push it. Push it in.
C. *(Crying)*
T. What do you see yourself doing now?
C. What I've done so many times before. *(Crying)* I have been so scared that I'll lose control.
T. This is in your imagination. She is not really here.
C. Yeah, but I don't even want to imagine it.
T. I know. Let's give it a try. Try it once. It'll be OK. Now maybe we can give it up. Go on. You can see your hand move. It is like something snaps in your head. You are not yourself anymore. It is not really you, because you wouldn't do that, but it is your body moving and your hands. Somebody's pushing. See

her face there. Really try to see her face. You see her face and you have the pencil and you can't control your hands. You want to, but you can't. You are not yourself. Something snaps in your mind and you see the pencil. You see the pencil moving into her face now. There it goes. Right in there. There it goes. Your hand shoved it right in there. Can you see that? Can you see your hand in there? See the pencil. You are holding it. It's stuck in her. See that vision. Imagine that scene. Your hand. It is not you because your are totally out of control; you have gone haywire. You have lost control. Somebody else is pushing your hand, it seems like. It is not your fault, but your hand takes the pencil and pushes it right into her face. Right into her face. Can you see that?

C. Uh-huh. (*Sobbing*)

T. See it again now. See it happen again. Back and forth. Go ahead, move that pencil. Move that pencil you have in your hand back and forth. In and out.

C. (*Sobbing*)

T. Go ahead. In and out. You are doing fine. You can see it. See it. Continue to see it. Stay with it. Stay with it. See it again. You are doing fine. See it again.

C. (*Sobbing*)

T. Again and again and again and again and again. In and out. In and out. In and out and she just lays there. You poke it in and out. In and out. Jab.

C. Ew.

T. Jab. Jab. See it. Over and over and over and over. Jabbing in and out. Jabbing in and out. Jab, jab, jab, jab, jab. It's like you've totally lost control. You have gone completely crazy. There's no control. Something has really gone haywire with your head. It's like your brain has just gone crazy and you keep on jabbing. Jab, jab, jab. Watch your hand with that pencil go right into her face. Hold the pencil up to her again and then just lose control of your hand. Move that pencil down closer and closer. It is about where you would normally stop. You stop for a minute and then your hand just keeps going. Just keeps going right in. Right in her face. You are moving it down again. You are where you usually stop now. You are horrified, but your hand just keeps poking it further into her. Right into her face. Right into her flesh. Right into her eyes. See the eyes now. Poke. She is looking at you. Jab, jab. Poking her, poking her. Pushing. Poking in and pulling out. Over and over and over and over again. It is like you are never going to stop.

C. (*Crying*)

T. See her face. She is looking at you again and you are walking by and you get the urge. You can't resist it. There is a pencil laying there. You grab that pencil and you go up to her. She is looking at you. Something snaps in your mind. You can't control yourself. You bring that pencil up to her. You know you won't hesitate this time. You jam it right into her eye. The other eye just keeps looking at you. You pull it out and you jab that eye. Your hand just moves and jabs it right into her eye. Do you see that?

C. Uh-huh.

T. See it again now. See it again. It's hard, but stay with it. Take that pencil. You have totally lost control. You can't control yourself. It's what you've always feared would happen. You lose control. You knew it would happen sooner or later. You would just lose control. You are not yourself. Something snaps, and you had that pencil as she is looking up at you, and you take that pencil and you feel yourself with all your force jamming that pencil right into her. Right into her. Then you jam it right into her eye. See it. See it going down into her eye. Feel yourself doing it. Feel your hand moving. Right into her eye. Then you jab it into her other eye. See it now. Keep imagining that scene. Let's just keep right on. Just see it over and over again. Stick right with that now. Just keep at it. You are doing fine. That's good. Keep doing it until it just becomes mechanical, automatic. Her face there, pulling the pencil out, sticking it in, pulling it out, sticking it in, pulling it out.

C. No. No. (*Crying*)

T. Keep seeing it. See the pencil. Feel it in your hand. You try to control it. You see her face there and you try to control it. You really try to control it. Hold the pencil right up to her. You see her eyes looking up at you. Closer and closer and closer to her eyes and then your hand just moves it right in her eye. Right into her eyes. See it again and again. In and out. In and out. See it. Can you see it going in? Can you feel your hands moving? You are doing fine. Put it right in there. Pay attention now to the sensations in your stomach, in your chest, and in your arms. The tightness in your head and face. Concentrate on those things a minute. Feel the scary feeling of what you are doing. The scary feeling of loss of control. See how you have lost control as you go in and out with that pencil. See it poking her in and out. You go in and out with that pencil. See it. The loss of control. See how you have lost control as you go in and out with that pencil. See it. Poking in and out. Feel those feelings. Feel anything you feel. Feel those feelings starting now to get stronger as you see yourself losing total control like a mad woman. Gone mad. You just feel it. Feel all those feelings. Let them go. Just continue to do this. In and out. In and out. You become almost like a mechanical person. Going in and out. In and out. No control. It's like somebody wound you up, like a clock is running in you. In and out. In and out. Over and over and over and over and over and over again. You have totally lost control. No contact with reality. You don't know what's going on around you. All you can see is that pencil and it goes in and out and in and out and in and out. You see it over and over and over and over. You can't control your hand. You are slashing into her face. What kind of thoughts run through your mind as you watch that going in and out, feeling your hand do it?

C. (*Sobbing*)

T. A mechanical hand. You finally did it. You finally went totally berserk. Now that hand just works by itself. You couldn't stop it if you wanted to. Just continue and continue and continue and continue. You can see it now. It's very clear. Let those thoughts go through your mind.

C. I'm thinking it's her fault. (*Crying*)

T. See her face there and tell her that. Say, "It's your fault that I am feeling like this . . . your fault."

C. (*Sobbing*) It's your fault.

T. See her face there and feel, feel it and really tell her.
C. Karen, this is all your fault.
T. It's all your fault.
C. It's not all her fault.
T. No, it's not *all* her fault, but right now feel it. Feel it right now. See her face and really see that it's her fault. Just for a few minutes. Feel that. Really feel that. Getting up in the morning, feeding her, being tied in the house. All that anxiety is her fault. And you tell her that. You tell her, "It's your fault." You go over to the dresser and you grab that pencil and you come down and you hold it to her eyes and you see her looking up at you. You see she is totally dependent on you. You've got to feed her and take care of her and stay home with her. You don't get to have any fun ever again. You don't get to go out. You are a mother now. You're just a mother. You have to take care of her all the time. You have no life of your own. It's her fault and you say, "It's your fault" and you plunge the pencil into her eyes. Tell her that. "It's your fault."
C. It's your fault. (*Sobbing*)
T. That's right, tell her again. You did this to me. I was doing fine until you came along. I had a good job, a good marriage, I was feeling good about myself and now look. I have all this fear and it's your fault. I don't want to be a mother. Tell her that.
C. But I do.
T. Tell her that anyway.
C. (*Sobbing*) I don't want to be a mother. I wish you would just go away.
T. Just go away. Leave me alone . . . tell her that. Leave me alone. Damn you . . . leave me alone. Feel what you are feeling now because what you are feeling now is really good. Feel it. Feel it. Clinch your jaw at all of this and get angry at it all. Get angry at the whole scene. Get angry at her. Feel it. It's time to. It's time to say, "the hell with all of this." What other thoughts run through your mind as you see your hand doing that?
C. I just hear her screaming.
T. You hear her screaming, crying, and what else?
C. I'm thinking about what's going to happen when they find out I have done all of this.
T. We know what's going to happen. It will be the end of you. Feel what you are feeling now. That's OK. Feel it. Clinch your teeth. Look at her. Feel the anger. Put it out. You do feel anger and you feel scared.
C. (*Sobbing*)
T. Hold that pencil tight.* Now take the pencil with both hands. Get it and break that pencil. Feel it now as you break it. Break it.
C. (*Breaks pencil*)
T. That's right. Feel that.
C. (*Sobbing*)

*At this point the session was getting long; the next few images were used to reduce anxiety before ending the session. Marsha had to go through this scene many times before there was much reduction in her emotional response.

T. Feel yourself break that pencil. You're done. You've finished that job. You turn around and walk out of that room. Throw that pencil on the floor. Go ahead and throw that pencil on the floor.

C. (*Sobbing, throws pencil on floor*)

T. Now you feel a total release. Feel the release from all that. Now let it go. Stand there with that broken pencil. You go to all of the objects you've had now and you start busting them up. You are breaking them up one by one. Can you see that? Can you go through your house? Go through your house and find an object. What do you find?

C. A knife.

T. A knife. You take that knife and what do you do with it?

C. I see myself, like so many times before, take the knife and I would put it back in the drawer and I would slam the drawer shut.

T. OK, slam it shut. The knife jumps back out. You can't get rid of it.

C. (*Sobbing*) That's just it, I can't.

T. You can't get rid of that. It just keeps jumping back out at you. Take that knife and you have got superhuman strength. Superhuman strength comes over your body. You go to the door and you take that knife and you rear back and you throw the knife two hundred miles away. Throw it very hard. It soars away. You go and you get another knife. You take that and with superhuman strength you throw that two hundred miles away. Can you see that? Get a whole bunch of knives now. One after another you throw them way up into the clouds. Way far away. Lots of strength. Lots of strength. You are very powerful. You can feel the strength flowing into your body now. You take another knife and just throw it way up in the air. Far away. It hasn't even landed yet. It's still going further and further away. What else do you find around your house?

C. Pins. Straight pins.

T. What do you do with those?

C. Throw them away.

T. See yourself doing that. What else.

C. Hot water.

T. See the pan. You fill it up with hot boiling water and then you circle it over your head and throw it far, far away. Just continue to throw everything. Every pointed, sharp, and dangerous object there is. You can just destroy that whole house. OK, open your eyes.

C. (*Sobbing*)

T. How do you feel?

C. Tired.

T. Tired, that's good. Do you feel relieved?

C. Immediately, I found myself thinking about when you were telling me to throw all the stuff away that I would have to go back and have to do all those things to her that I had never done other than with the pencil. And would just have to do them all.

T. You felt like you should have to do them all?

C. Uh-huh. Wonder why?

T. Why do you think?
C. I don't know.
T. Do you feel like you would have to do it with the pencil, too, or with everything else.
C. With everything else.
T. All right, but would you have to do it with the pencil?
C. That did not flash through my mind, I guess because I had already done that.
T. Do you think you could ever do anything like that in real life?
C. (*Sobbing*) No. I don't know why it bothers me.
T. That's why it's important to go through it. To realize that you can imagine it without it bothering you.
C. I don't think I should even imagine it not bothering me. (*Sobbing*) Because, if I don't want to hurt her, why do I imagine things like that?
T. How do you think Karen is right now?
C. OK.
T. Do you think she is hurt by any of this?
C. No.
T. Then how does it hurt her to imagine things?
C. (*Sobbing*) I didn't used to imagine things like that around people. If I did, I didn't realize.
T. If imagining it would help you stop from being tempted to bring stuff up to her face, wouldn't you be helping her? She's not hurt by it. We feel that going over these things over and over and over again will reduce these feelings you're having until you finally let yourself really feel it all. And you feel the anger, too.
C. Uh-huh. The feeling of actually wanting to do it is there. It's just the thought of doing. I have actually tried to get the feeling of like I wanted to do it.
T. You were trying to test your loss of control to see if you will lose control. And what we're saying is . . . OK. Sometimes you lose control. Just go ahead and feel what it's like. It's a fantasy. Fantasies won't hurt you and they won't hurt her.
C. But why do I have that thought?
T. I think that you have these thoughts of doing it, but you have never been able to go ahead and do it all the way and be done with it. You can't in real life. The only way you can do it is in fantasy. Before you can be done with it maybe you can imagine all of it several times. It gets to be very routine. Let me tell you about a fantasy I used to have that I thought was horrible . . .

Marsha was encouraged to practice the scene at home as much as possible and to not engage in the checking behavior. However, if she did engage in the checking behavior, she was to call the therapist to help her work through the guilt (this also served as a suicide precaution).

One of Marsha's problems was her inability to be assertive enough to express negative feelings towards anyone, much less her child. We saw this inability to express anger as one of the main causes of her disorder. Thus, becoming more assertive was a goal of therapy. To help her with this, we used the technique of *priming* described in Chapter 4. Recall that the procedure involves taking a past event that has aroused the inhibited emotion in the patient and having him or her relive that event in imagination. Often these scenes are only tangentially related to the central theme of therapy, but they will help the patient to express the inhibited emotion in front of another person (the therapist). Marsha had rarely expressed anger in front of another person and priming made it easier for her to show anger more relevant to her problem later on in therapy. To obtain material for the priming scene, Marsha was asked to tell us about the last time she had felt "very angry." The following transcript is part real event and part fantasy relating to an interaction Marsha had with a doctor.

T. That doctor doesn't like you at all. You say that sometimes you are a bitch. "You are. You are just self-centered, righteous, you don't care about anyone and I don't care about anyone either. I don't care about you, I don't care about that kid." Why don't you look at the doctor now and tell him he can just go to hell.
C. Why don't you just go to hell?
T. Tell him again. Make a fist with your hand and bang on the chair and tell him that.
C. Just go to hell. Just leave me alone.
T. Tell him again. See his face. He hates you. He doesn't care about you. He made you worse. You are in this fix because of him. Tell him to go to hell.
C. Why don't you just go to hell. It's all your fault. You didn't help me a bit.
T. He just laughs. He says, "That's right. I didn't help you and I didn't want to help you. I am glad you're sicker. Just what I wanted." And you just make a fist and you say, "You son of a bitch, I hate you." Tell him that.
C. You son of a bitch, I hate you.
T. Then you take his feet and you kick them off where he has got them propped up. Get them off his pedestal. Kick them off. Real hard. See yourself doing that?
C. Uh-huh.
T. Kick them off. Real hard. See it. See it there.
C. I am.
T. He says, "You self-centered bitch, get out of my office." And you say, "I'll be glad to get out of your office after I tell you what your problem is." Tell him that.
C. I will be glad to get out of your office after I tell you what your problem is.
T. "You're self-centered and you are a lousy physician and I am going to sue the hell out of you." Tell him that.
C. You're self-centered. You're a lousy physician and I am going to sue the hell out of you.
T. Tell him that with some feeling. Really feel it. See his face there. You have been suffering and suffering. It's his fault. And he doesn't care about you. He doesn't care about your baby or what might happen to your baby or you or your family. He just wants your money and to throw some pills your way. He doesn't care about you at all. Tell him that *he's* the self-centered one.

C. You are self-centered. All you care about is the money that I send in here every week always telling me, "I want to see you again, I want to see you again."

T. That's right, tell him.

C. Rather than saying, "I think you're getting better or I think you are making progress or the time of day or anything."

T. "I told you that because I wanted you to know that you were a sick-o. That's why I told you that." You just look at him and you say, "You bastard, you are harming people and you have harmed me. You have no right to practice medicine." Tell him that.

C. You have no right to practice medicine. You have done me a lot of harm and I am sure you have done a lot more people a lot of harm. In fact, I know now there is a woman who was seeing you and I think that was a lot of her problem . . . you messed her up, too.

T. Suddenly, he jumps up and says, "You have no right to talk to me about that." He slaps you across the face. He really like flips out and he jumps up and he slaps you across the face. Can you see that?

C. Uh-huh.

T. He's big. He comes right at you and you see that hand coming down and he slaps you right across the face and you feel a stinging on your face. It kind of startles you. Then he takes his other hand and he slaps you across the face again very hard. He slaps you again and you are very startled and it kind of throws you back and you realize he really does hate you. He really hates you and he takes his hand now and you see this big man in front of you and his hand is coming down and you see his eyes glaring at you and his teeth clinched together. He's really angry at you now, he really hates you. He's very big and he takes that hand out and he slaps you across your face again. Do you feel that? See him now. The pain and shock of it. Then he takes his big hands and he shoves you back and you fall over the chair and he kicks you and he says, "I hate you. You have no right to call me that. You son of a bitch." He just keeps kicking you and throwing you against the wall. He throws you up against the wall. You feel that wall slam up against your back and you go in a heap down in the floor and he kicks you some more. He kicks you some more. How do you feel when this is going on?

C. I scream, "Stop, leave me alone, let me get out of here. You're insane."

T. You do that, "Stop, stop!" He won't stop. He just keeps kicking you. He goes crazy. He just keeps kicking you and slapping you and hitting you and you see all of it. That hand coming at you. He is throwing you against the wall . . . The pain of it. You see it all. You see it all and you realize that he is not going to let you out of that office. He's not. He's going to kill you right there in the office. He keeps slapping you and hitting you. He goes crazy. You feel the blood on your body now. And suddenly, the helplessness changes. You feel something snap in your brain. It's like you are not yourself anymore. You just get superhuman strength now and you just look up at him and he is towering up above you and you say, "You bastard. You ugly bastard."

C. You bastard. You ugly bastard.

T. You look at him and you see the hate he has for you and how he has hurt you. It goes through your mind how he is hurting you, but that's the least of it. How he has hurt you in the past and on purpose he was hurting you. All the suffering you did. The crying and the pain you have undergone. It's all due to him. He towers above you and you think of all that pain you've undergone as he is kicking you while you are down. Walking on you while you are on the floor. He doesn't care about you at all. You say, "You bastard." Then you jump up and something snaps in your mind and you have superhuman strength and you say, "You bastard." You take your fist and you slam it into his mouth and he is startled. He didn't expect that. Can you see that? Why don't you take your hand and really move it into the air now. Can you see his face?

C. Uh-huh.

T. That's right. Hit him again. Harder. Feel the fist hit his face. Let it go right into his face. He is really big so you've got to hit him again. When you hit him say, "You bastard."

C. (*Crying*) You bastard, why did you do this to me . . .

T. It's your fault. Why did you let me suffer so? Hit him again. You're doing fine. See his face. Come on. He made you suffer like that. Feel it. Good. Everytime you see his face in your mind you hit him again. See his face there. There is still kind of a smile and a smirk on his face.

C. Yeah, he always had a smirk.

T. Right, always had that smirk. See it. See that smirk he always had. Hit it. Wipe that smirk off his face. Wipe that smirk off his face. Then he trips. He trips because you have been hitting him, but he is still smirking up at you. So you start kicking him. You walk on him like he has walked on you. Walk on him. Jump up and down on him now. Really stomp him. Can you see that?

C. I can see him down there, but I can't . . .

T. Take your heel and put it up to his face and grind it right into his mouth. See that smirk? He was happy you were suffering. See him gag.

C. Why would he want to be happy though?

T. Just feel it for the next minutes. It doesn't have to be true. Right now you see his smirk. You see his smirk and know that right now in this scene he hates you and he has been hitting you and walking on you. You feel the blood coming down from your own mouth. He has beaten you to a pulp. There is no way you can get out of that room and you had to hit him. Something snaps in your mind. It's like you're not yourself now. He's on the ground still smiling and he's about ready to get up and hit you some more. You take your heel and you slam it into him. See him down there. Slam your heel into him. He deserves it. It's his fault that your're suffering. He deserves it. Can you see that? Slam your heel into his face. That's right, that's good. Feel the pressure. See him gag. Slam it down again. It's his fault that you've suffered so much. It's his fault. Good. How do you feel now?

C. Tired and upset. Drained.

T. Cue in on that tired feeling. See his face there. Step on it.

C. I keep on saying, "Why, why, why? Why did you do this?"

T. He says, "Because I hate people like you and your petty little gripes and bitches. You don't know what real trouble is." Look down at him and tell him, "You're sick. I don't have to take anymore of you."
C. You're sick. You're sicker than I am. I don't have to take anymore of this.
T. Feel it. He's sick and crazy and what he did was sick and crazy. He did it to you. You have every right to feel that way. It's true. Look at him. Pound him again and look at him. Come on and pound him. Come on and feel it. Yeah, feel it. Pound him and pound him. Reach down now and take his hands and put them around his throat. Go ahead. Feel his throat. You squeeze his throat. Feel it. Squeeze. Look at it. Look at him. Squeeze on that neck for what he did to you. You're going to fix it so he won't do it to you or anybody else.*

The course of therapy was variable. Marsha found it difficult to practice scenes at home, especially when she was having a "good day," preferring instead to avoid the thoughts altogether. When this happens, we try to contract with the client to practice the scenes routinely and at specified times during the day. If this is still not effective, it may he helpful to tape record sessions and ask the client to use the tape to stimulate homework sessions. We did both with Marsha. However, this latter method is to be avoided, if possible, as it does not allow the patient to embellish the material with more personally meaningful imaginal scenes.

Another problem in Marsha's therapy was that there was little generalization from one obsessional thought to another. When she learned to control or extinguish the anxiety associated with one thought (e.g., putting a pointed object into the child's eyes), she would switch to one of her other obsessions (e.g., burning the child). Each thought had to be flooded individually.

Marsha's concern that the child would pull scalding water over on her may have been more significant than the other obsessions since it represented an earlier childhood experience. What follows is a transcript of the scene we used to extinguish that fear.

T. What do you see?
C. I see Karen.
T. Are you in your house?
C. Uh-huh.
T. How come you're in your house.
C. Don't know.
T. Let's take a trip around your house with Karen. Where are you?
C. In the kitchen.
T. Is your kitchen divided off from your dining room?
C. No. I have a combination.
T. Do you have a dining area?

*The supportive therapist–client interactions that followed scene presentation have been omitted; these interactions, however, are essential for successful therapy.

C. I have a formal dining room and a dining area in the kitchen.
T. OK. A formal dining area and that's off from the kitchen and then a dining area in the kitchen?
C. Yes.
T. Can you walk from the kitchen into the dining room?
C. Uh-huh.
T. OK. Imagine you're doing that. Go by the dining area when you're doing that.
C. Uh-huh.
T. You go through the kitchen by the counters and stove. You go on into the dining room. Can you walk out of that room into another room?
C. Into the living room. It has an archway.
T. Into the living room. Is it a one-story?
C. Uh-huh.
T. Do you go down the hallway to the bedroom?
C. Yes. From the living room either go back into the dining room or into the foyer and go back into the den. The den is right off from the kitchen. It doesn't have a door ledge, just an opening. Go down the hall into the bedroom. The bedrooms are all down the hall.
T. Three bedrooms?
C. Uh-huh.
T. OK. Walk back down the hall. Imagine yourself walking. Holding onto her hand. She toddles along. Is she a pretty good walker now?
C. Yes.
T. Gets around good and is into a lot of things?
C. Yes. Lots of times she'll take your finger and lead you around the house.
T. OK. I want you to imagine now that you sit down and start to watch television and she goes on and plays. You kind of keep an eye on her. You see her playing around. She goes into the kitchen. Can you see that?
C. Yes.
T. Imagine that you are there now. You are really there. You're sitting there and you see her toddling around. If you try real hard, you can really be there now. Can you see her walk into the kitchen? What would you do or how would you feel?
C. It would be two different ways. If I am not cooking or anything like that, I would just let her go in there and I would feel fairly comfortable. If I was cooking, I would go to get her or tell her to come back and come stay with me. I would probably have to go get her. She has a table and chairs in the den and and I keep a lot of toys in there.
T. I want you to see her now. You see her walking into the kitchen and you are cooking. I want you to imagine that you tell her to come back and she doesn't come back. So you get up and you come into the kitchen and just as you come into the kitchen you see her reach up and grab boiling water that's on the stove. Can you see that?
C. Uh-huh.
T. She pulls it down and you can see it come down on her. Feel that now. You start to scream. You come over to get her and she's burnt badly. She's crying

and she's screaming. You rush to her as fast as you can to wash her off with cold water. You get her into the bathtub to put cold water on her. You can't get the water on. The water won't turn on. She's screaming and crying. You can't cool her off at all. You see her starting to get red now. Red and she feels hot. She's crying, "Mama, Mama, it hurts." See it. A whole pot of boiling water. Then she starts to just black out. She doesn't cry anymore. You try to shake her awake, but she is still out. You go to the phone to call for some help. You call the doctor and he sends an ambulance to come and get her. You can see this. The ambulance comes up to the front of the house. You are holding her in your arms; she's not moving. Feel that fear you feel right now. That warm body and she's just lying there. She's really hurt badly. She's burned all over. She's still breathing, but she's burned all over. Feel it. They take her from you and they put her into the ambulance and drive away. You get into your car and go after it. You get to the hospital. You go into the hospital. You can smell that hospital. You can feel and see the people. You go into the room where she is. She's all wrapped up and she's had a special bath. You talk to the doctors about her. They don't know if she's going to pull through this or not. See it. She is burned all over her body. They ask you what happened. Then you tell them your story. You sit there and you wait all through the night. You watch her and early that next morning you see her and she hasn't moved. She isn't breathing anymore. She dies. You see her there all burned and puffed up. Distorted, ugly face. You have to face your family and your friends and you wonder what they will think. See her there. Look at this. It happened again. You thought you had learned by your experience not to let this happen again. You let it happen again. That's what happened. You didn't control the situation. You are not a good mother. You feel the guilt. You could've stopped her if you had been more involved. Instead of sitting there yelling, you should have gone after her right away. You knew the hot water was there. You could've stopped her, but you didn't. You were in the wrong. You know it. What kind of thoughts go through your mind when you realize that your baby is dead?

C. Unbearable pain. (*Crying*)

T. What kind of thoughts do you have?

C. I feel guilty. It's like you said. I could have actually prevented it. I didn't intentionally do it.

One significant aspect to Marsha's treatment was to give her "permission" to have angry thoughts. We stressed the fact that thoughts don't hurt anyone and that everybody had hostile urges towards their children. This rational-emotive ploy was not entirely successful, but helped some. A variety of antidepressant medications was also used, but none appeared to affect the obsessions. Toward the end of therapy a small amount of Haldol (25 mg per day) may have been useful.

After 22 treatment sessions, Marsha complained little of thoughts. We followed her for two years and saw her briefly on a monthly basis for an additional six months. Her main concern during the early follow-up period was whether or not to have a second child. Eventually, she did have a second child and had no problems with obsessional thoughts toward the child. The child is two years old at this writing.

Case Study 2

Steve was a 35-year-old single man with a severe obsessive-compulsive disorder. He was obsessed with being able to recall and recreate in his mind everything that was said to him and felt out of control and doubtful of his sanity when unable to do so. Compulsive rituals filled his day. For example, it took him three hours to perform his morning routine. Each activity, from making his bed to removing his pajamas and going to the toilet, was performed according to complex time-consuming rituals. We hypothesized that lying behind the obsessive thoughts and compulsive rituals was fear of losing control, of expressing his anger (particularly toward his parents), and of going crazy. In fact, he never expressed even mild anger. We also believed that a strong fear of abandonment—of being left to fend for himself with none of his needs met—inhibited anger expression, as did an overdeveloped sense of guilt regarding anger expression (his parents had severely punished any overt expression of anger).

Steve had been hospitalized numerous times in the past and was often diagnosed as schizophrenic. However, we felt that he was a severely incapacitated obsessive compulsive. One of us treated him as an inpatient by using both implosive scenes and *in vivo* exposure. A complete transcript of the fifth implosive therapy session follows, and illustrates a scene aimed at extinguishing the fear of anger expression and of loss of control. The scene also touches on strong guilt cues and acceptance of conscience. Additionally, at this point in the therapy, it was felt that some resistance to therapy had been built-up, with the client fearing that the therapy would itself drive him crazy. Consequently, an attempt was made to reduce this resistance by extinguishing the fear that the therapy would drive him crazy. Homework instructions for practicing the implosive scenes and for using response prevention to disrupt a compulsive ritual were also provided.

T. How have you been since Friday?

C. Well, um, I don't really know. I don't seem able to go back and recreate these things like I have been. That's making me a little shakey, I think.

T. You mean you're not as able to recreate what's happened to you?

C. No. You've kind of put doubts in my mind. You know, before I knew exactly and I could go back and recreate, but now because of these doubts I'm beginning to wonder.

T. And when you wonder if you're able to recreate it exactly, does it bother you as much?

C. Yes, it bothers me. Because I was always so under control.
T. Um hum. And you interpret not being able to remember as being less in control.
C. Right. Like, for instance, when you came to get me and I was smoking. You know I go through this smoking ritual, and when I go back to recreate that, because I didn't expect to see you, you kind of threw me off.
T. So you had to think about it afterwards, decide if you handled your cigarette properly and so on?
C. I had to kind of think about it before I could put it out.
T. On Friday you said you were no longer smoking it to the last puff, but just throwing it out earlier.
C. That's right.
T. Has it gone back to the old way?
C. No, it hasn't.
T. So when you threw your cigarette out when I was down there, that was not the last puff?
C. No.
T. It was pretty far down, but it wasn't the last puff. And you're having doubts in your mind as to whether you are able to recreate things as well since we started therapy. And it still scares you to have those doubts.
C. Yes. It does.
T. Is there any other thing that you've noticed? Any other changes?
C. Uh, yes, I seem to have almost forgotten how to do things. Like today when I was dressing, and making the bed and so on, you know I go through, well, I don't think it's exactly a ritual, it's more a routine. But I have to stop and think about how I've—I guess maybe it is a ritual because I have to stop and think about how I've always done things.
T. Feeling that you need to do it that way this time.
C. Um hum, yeah.
T. Anything else on your mind?
C. Well, no, except that I just kind of get in a panic when I can't remember something. And I don't seem to be able to focus on a conversation.
T. Because you're trying to remember something?
C. Um hum. Because I'm trying to remember something. Like, it's kind of like I know what I know, but I have doubts. Like I know that I was smoking when you came to get me, but later if I go back and try to think about it, I won't be able to. I'll just have—well, not exactly—doubts. I still know, but I'll have to think about it.
T. Um hum. And it still matters to you a lot to get it right?
C. Um hum.
T. OK. How many times were you able to do the homework scene?
C. I believe about 6 or 7.
T. OK. That's about twice a day.
C. Um hum.
T. And how did that go?
C. Um, I think I was better able to put myself in it rather than looking on.

T. Good. How much better were you able to do it?

C. Well, it took some work. It took doing it a few times. But I think that the last 3 times I was better able to.

T. Um hum. So, for example, in the scene where they put you in the hospital and strap you down, you said before that you were kind of looking on in that scene. And were you able to get to the point where you actually felt yourself being strapped down and saw what you would see in that vision?

C. Um hum.

T. Well, good. You know, I've had you rate these scenes from 0 to 100 with 100 being terror and 0 being calm. You rated that scene in the office as 90, I believe. Would you rate it as it was during your homework, perhaps the first time or two and the last time or two?

C. It went from about 85 down to about 70, I guess.

T. OK. How are you feeling right now?

C. I feel a little bit panicky because, as I said, when you came down I was smoking. And I'm not sure I did it, you know, the way I usually do it.

T. Um hum. Which part of the ritual do you think you haven't done?

C. Well, let's see. Even though I don't smoke it down all the way, I still think about the fact that this is going to be the last puff. And I just throw it in the ash tray. And I know that I just threw it in the ash tray, because that's just—I just never put them out any other way.

T. But is that the part you have a little doubt about?

C. No. The part that I have doubts about is whether or not that was really going to be my last puff, because, you know, you were waiting and everything.

T. But you really didn't have enough time to decide because I came down and hurried you a little. My presence hurried you.

C. Well, just your presence, yeah.

T. Um huh. So you're not sure if you really decided whether that was your last puff or not?

C. Yeah.

T. Can you close your eyes and picture that? Only this time when you run through it, I want you to picture that it really wasn't your last puff. It was maybe the second to the last puff, or the third from the last, and you still threw it away. You're sitting there on the ward facing the nurses' desk there and you're smoking your cigarette. And then you see Dr. Shipley come in and he comes over to you and says, "It's time for your session." And then you think, it's not your last puff yet, and you take another puff. Dr. Shipley starts to walk away, then he walks back again and you take another puff. But you realize that it's still not your last puff. And then I want you to see yourself; it's not your last puff, you haven't finished, but Dr. Shipley is standing there; he's looking down at you. You see him looking down at you?

C. Um hum.

T. And he looks impatient. I want you to really see that he really looks impatient. He's a busy man, you get that feeling, and he is not going to wait for you. And he's really upset—you can tell—maybe he's had a bad day or something, but he's upset with you. He's really upset with you and he just thinks that cigarette ritual is silly. And you know that and you feel this great pressure to get moving and get up there. But you didn't take your last puff, you didn't take that last puff yet, you know you didn't. You know that and yet there he is and he wants you to hurry up. He doesn't say anything, but you know that, you can tell. He's impatient. He's kind of pacing and he's looking down at you. He's in a hurry. So you take that cigarette and you toss it in the ashtray without taking the last puff. And then you get up and you go with him. And it's still on your mind. You didn't take that last puff. You didn't take that last puff, and there's no doubt about it. You didn't take it. You feel that?

C. Uh hum.

T. What kind of thoughts go through your mind?

C. Um, well, just, I'm just frightened because I can't go back and recreate exactly how it happened.

T. It doesn't frighten you that you're sure that you didn't take the last puff?

C. No, that doesn't frighten me.

T. It would be frightening if you were kind of in doubt about it?

C. Yeah, one thing is the fact that even though you were standing there, I didn't. So that I guess it would be closer to the last puff. I did take one more puff while you were still standing there.

T. But you're not really sure, even though it was closer to the last puff than if you had come right away. You're not really sure if that was the last puff.

C. Right.

T. And you're not sure if you made your mind up whether that was the last puff.

C. Right.

T. And there's some doubt in your mind about that. A lot of doubt, as a matter of fact. I want you to feel that. There's a lot of doubt about that. You can't really decide. And no matter how many times you go through it in your mind, I want you to picture this now, no matter how many times, you'll never be sure. That doubt will always be there. Do you feel that? (*Client nods*) There's no way for you to ever know. That doubt will always be there. You never will know whether you actually consciously took that last puff or not, or if it was just one of the last puffs. You'll never be able to know. I want you to feel that. Never be able, that doubt will always be in your mind. It's eating at you. Eating at you. You can't get it out of your mind. Did you take the last puff or not? And what does that doubt mean?

C. It, it frightens me.

T. It means that you're slipping, doesn't it? It means that you're slipping. Your mind is going.

C. Slipping.

T. That's right. And you're trying to . . .

C. (*Interrupting*) Well, I don't know that it means that. It just means that I have to work harder at recreating it.

T. Right. But I want you to feel that the harder you work, the harder you work, the more doubt that comes into your mind.

C. Um hum.

T. It makes it worse. The harder you work, the more doubt, the more doubt comes into your mind. You're not sure if that was the last puff or not. You just can't decide. And you think of it one way, and you think of it the other way, and you think of it in between those ways, and you're not sure. They're all equally probable. And the doubt is there. And then it comes to you that you're slipping. Your mind is going. And you remember other things that you can't remember, that you can't recreate. And it's happening more and more, isn't it? More and more that you can't keep that straight. You remember other incidents and the doubt is cumulative. It just all adds up, because every little incident, all of them unresolved and all of them you have to think about and you can't physically do it anymore. You just don't have enough hours in the day to figure it out and you can't anyway. The more time you spend, the more confused you get. The more confused and doubtful. And you realize, you feel this now, you realize that you're slipping. Your mind is going. Do you get that feeling?

C. Yes, but it's very, very uncomfortable.

T. I want you to stay with that though, really stay with that. Remember that you can't remember what happened with that cigarette. Not only that, but you can't remember other things. It's like the therapy that Dr. Shipley is doing with you is really driving you crazy. It really's going to make you crazy. I want you to get that feeling.

C. That's exactly how it feels.

T. That's right, that's right. That's exactly how it feels. I want you to feel it right now.

C. I do.

T. Right. That therapy is going to drive you crazy. And each time you go in . . .

C. It's already beginning to.

T. That's right. It's driving you crazy already, and each time it gets worse and worse and worse. And I want you to picture that you're back on the ward now after about the 15th session, and you can't remember anything. And you're wandering around like a zombie now. And you try to remember and you can't remember about putting your fork down or not, you can't remember whether you pulled your pants up right in the morning, you can't remember anything. You can't remember the last 25 times about your cigarette, whether you threw it in or put it in, whether you took the last puff, you can't remember. And you try to think of all of those times. But you can't because that therapy is making you crazy. It's made your mind just slip away, a little bit at a time. Away, away, away, and pretty soon it's just a shadow of its former self. You can't remember how to make your bed in the morning. You can't remember how to take your shower. How to pull up your pants. You can't remember how to eat. You can't remember how to relate. You don't know how to do anything. You have no being. You just can't remember anything. One big doubt after another. And you can't get reassurance from anybody. Nobody will tell you, will they? Nobody will tell you whether you did it or not. You can't remember yourself. And you feel yourself slipping. I want you to feel that now, can you feel that?

C. Yes.

T. That's right. Just stay with it now. You feel yourself slipping and your mind is going. Stay with that feeling now, just stay with it. Your mind is going and you're going crazy, and you're going crazy and it's because of that therapy. It's because of that therapy and you're slipping away. You're slipping away. You can't remember whether you took the last puff. You can't remember whether you put that fork on the table or not. I want you to feel that now. You can't remember it. Stay with it. You can't remember it. And you feel yourself starting to shake. And your mind is slipping. And you feel it and you know it, that it's slipping away. It's slipping away.

C. Oh, oh. (*Shaking*)

T. And it's slipping away. And you can't hold it togehter. And you're afraid you're going to go crazy. Really crazy! And you feel yourself getting closer and closer to being really crazy now. Steve, your mind is slipping away. Your mind is slipping away and you can't remember whether you took the last puff. You can't remember whether you took the last puff. You can't remember. You can't remember. It's all doubt. You can't remember about making the bed and how to do it and how to take a shower. You can't remember that. You can't remember it. You can't. You know you probably did it wrong. You probably made your bed wrong. And you took your shower wrong this morning. And you put your fork in the wrong place and ate wrong and put your dishes away wrong. And you smoked your cigarette all wrong. For the last week now, it's all been wrong, wrong, wrong. And you can't remember whether you did it wrong or right, but somehow you feel it was wrong, improper. And you feel your mind slipping away, slipping away. That's right. And you start to shake all over; as your mind slips away, so does your body. So does your body and your mind can't control your body, it can't control your thoughts, and it's just slipping away now. You feel that?

C. Yes, yes.

T. Really stay with it now. You feel it just slipping away. Slipping away. That's right and it just gets worse and worse and worse. And it's because of that therapy. I want you to feel that, it's because of that therapy. And you feel that tension throughout your body. The tension and the shaking and the nausea. And you feel that it just makes you crazier and crazier, crazier and crazier. Do you feel that?

C. Yes. (*Tearful*)

T. Stay with that now. What kind of thoughts run through your mind as you feel your doubts and you feel that you've done things improperly? What kind of thoughts run through your mind?

C. The improper part doesn't bother me so much, but the feeling that I'm going crazy.

T. And what kind of thoughts, as you think you're going crazy, what kind of thoughts run through your mind?

C. I feel that I really am. (*Shaking*)

T. That you really are going crazy. And what will happen when you really do go crazy?

C. I don't know.

T. But it will be pretty bad. You don't know what it is, but it'll be bad, won't it?

C. Yes.

T. Right. It'll be pretty bad. You're not sure what it is—that's the worse part, not knowing. Not knowing what would happen. Not knowing, but fearing it'll be pretty bad. And after you're crazy, nobody will care for you at all. They'll all reject you, won't they?

C. (*Sobbing*)

T. Won't they?

C. Yes.

T. That's right. They'll hate you, 'cause you'll do crazy things. You'll do crazy things. And your mind will just fly here and there and you won't be able to stop it. You won't be able to control it. You won't be able to remember. You won't be able to keep yourself calm and functional. You won't be able to make your bed or take your shower even. You won't be able to feed yourself even. (*Client sobs*) You can't remember. You really have doubts. And then you can't remember about making your bed, did you do that the right way or not? And not getting dressed, you have doubts about that. I want you to feel that. You have doubts about getting dressed. Can you feel that?

C. Yes.

T. What doubts do you have about that?

C. Um, well no, I can't say that I do feel that.

T. I want you to be not sure about whether you got dressed the right way. Whether you washed the right way. Whether you ate the right way. Especially whether you put your dinner tray away wrong. You put your fork down in the wrong place. Maybe you did or maybe you didn't. You don't know. You can't keep your mind straight. You can't remember. I want you to feel that now. You can't remember. You can't remember anything now. And then your mind snaps. Your mind snaps, it does. I want you to feel that. Your mind snaps. You can't remember. And you go crazy. You go crazy. And what do you do?

C. (*Sob*) I don't know.

T. What do you do?

C. I don't know.

T. But you go crazy. Your mind goes. Your mind goes and you start screaming and yelling. And you know what you yell? You yell, "I hate you." You go crazy and you yell, "I hate you." See yourself now, you go crazy. You can't remember. And the stress and the strain of that therapy was just too much for you and you go completely crazy. Because you can't remember any of these things and you go crazy. You go crazy and you yell, "I hate you." "I hate you." And somebody comes up to you and says, "Steve, what's the matter?" And you say, "I hate you." Somebody else says, "What's going on?" and you turn to him and you see his face and you say, "I hate you." And you just go crazy. You start walking around telling every person you meet that you hate him. Do you see that?

C. Um hum. (*Feeble and quavery*)

T. I want you to walk up to somebody now, who is it? See somebody there.

C. Oh, I guess, Carl.

T. Yeah, there's Carl, right there. You see him.

C. Um hum.

T. He's just standing there. He's not even doing anything. And you walk up to him and you look him right in the eye, and see Carl right in your mind's eye now, and feel yourself; you see Carl and you're crazy now. You walk up to him and you say, "I hate you." See him and say that.

C. I hate you.

T. Right. And then you walk up to somebody else, and you see him. And you tell him the same thing.

C. I hate you.

T. And then somebody else.

C. I hate you!

T. That's right. Then you walk up to Dr. Shipley and you see him and you look up and you say, "I hate you."

C. I hate you.

T. That's right. Then you come up to somebody else now, Sue, you see Sue and you walk up to her and tell her that.

C. I hate you.

T. That's right. You tell everybody, "I hate you. I hate you. I hate you. I hate you." And you walk up to somebody else, somebody else, who's that?

C. Um, Pam.

T. Yeah. You tell her now.

C. I hate you.

T. You see her and tell her again.

C. I hate you!

T. That's right. Tell her again.

C. I hate you!!

T. And then you start swinging at them. You start swinging at them. You walk up to Pam again. You walk up to her and you say, "I hate you."

C. I hate you.

T. And then you take your hand and you hit her with it. You take your hand and you hit Pam right across the face. You say, "I hate you" and then you hit her. "I hate you," and you hit her again. You see that. I hate you and you hit her again. I hate you and you hit her again. And then you go up and there comes Dr. Shipley again, and you go up to him and you say, "I hate you." Say that.

C. I hate you.

T. See him there again. Say, "I hate you!"

C. I hate you!

T. And then you swing at him. And you hit him. Again and again and again and you kick him. And you're crazy now and you've got superhuman strength. Superhuman strength and you just hit him again and again and again and again and you push him to the ground now and you kick him. You kick him and you jump up and down on him and you keep saying, "I hate you, I hate you, I hate you, I hate you," and you jump on him and you kick his face. You kick his face. And you kick him in the groin now, and you just jump on him and spit on him and hit him and kick him and claw him. You see that now, you just destroy him and all that time you see his face and you say, "I hate, I hate you, I hate you." And then you pick up his body and you just throw it against the wall. You pick his body up and you're superhuman, do you see that?

C. Um hum.

T. You pick his body up, you're really crazy now. And he's unconscious and bleeding and you throw him against the wall. And he slides down against the wall. And he just lays there in a heap. And then you go get some other people. And you beat them up. You see that now. You've got some others? *(Client nods)* And you hit them and claw them and jump on them and destroy them. You just destroy them. And you rip them apart. And you throw them against the wall, Steve, you just throw them against the wall. And then you get somebody else. Somebody else and you're really crazy now, you're really wigged out, and you just go crazy. You just go crazy and all you want to do is kill. That's what you want to do. That's all you want to do is KILL, KILL, KILL! And you just start killing people. You just start destroying people now. You're killing them, one after another. Do you see that? Do you see that?

C. Yes. *(Feeble and crying)*

T. See it now. Stay with it. Stay with it. You see that. You're killing people. You're killing people, aren't you? Again and again and again.

C. *(Loud sobs)*

T. You're killing them. Yes, you are. You're killing them. You see that. And you walk up to them and you say, "I hate you! I hate you, I hate you!" And then you hit them and kick them and claw them and jump on them and throw them around the room. And you've got superhuman strength. Your mind has slipped. It's gone and you've gone crazy. You couldn't remember where you put that cigarette. You couldn't remember about that fork. You couldn't remember about the tray or getting dressed or making your bed and then you go crazy. You go crazy and you start killing people, don't you? You start killing people. And you go up to another one and you say, "I hate you. I hate you." See another one. Who's there now?

C. Mary.

T. There's Mary. And you go up and you say, "I hate you, Mary." Say that.

C. I hate you, Mary.

T. And you take her and you hit her. You see that? You hit her. And you hit again and again and again. You hit her. You take Mary and you destroy her. You destroy her and she's bleeding now. You throw her against the wall. There's a whole heap of bodies over there. And you kill her, you kill her. And then you go up to Dr. Smith. You go up to Dr. Smith and you say, "I hate you, I hate you." Tell him that now.

C. I hate you.

T. That's right. "I hate you" and then you kill him. You see yourself hitting him now, hitting him again and again and again and again and again and again . . .

C. *(Interrupting)* I don't know how much more I can take.

T. You're doing fine. Just stay with it; you just stay with it. You take him and you kill him and you throw him over next to Dr. Shipley over there with Mary and everybody. And you kill and kill and kill and kill. Do you see that? You've just gone crazy. You just go crazy. Your mind slips. Your mind slips and you go crazy. You go really stark raving mad now. And you just start killing everybody, everybody that comes. You just take them one at a time and you rip them apart. And you kill them. You kill them. You kill everybody. Everybody. Some other people come up to you now and you tell them. "I hate you. I hate you." Tell them that.

C. I hate you.

T. Tell them again.

C. I hate you!

T. And then you hit them. You hit them and you kill them. Do you see that?

C. Um hum.

T. You kill them, too, don't you?

C. Um hum.

T. And then what do you do? You've killed everybody on the ward now, everybody on the ward, you've killed them all. And they're all lying on the floor against the wall. And you look at all of them. You look at all of them and you tell them, "I hate you! I hate everybody! I hate you!" You see that? And then you go outside and you go home. You go home now. You see that?

C. Uh hum.

T. And you're at home now. And you walk in, you see your mother there. See your mother?

C. Um hum.

T. She walks over. And you've got blood all over you. And she says, "Steve, what is going on?" And you look at her. You look at her and you know she's the one that made you crazy. She's the one. Maybe she didn't mean to, but she's the one who really did it. I want you to feel that.

C. (*Sobbing*)

T. She's the one. When you were a little kid, you couldn't protect yourself; she destroyed your brain then. That's when she did it. And you look at her and you tell her, "I hate you!" You see her there and you tell her, "I hate you!"

C. I hate you!

T. That's right. You say, "Mother, I hate you."

C. Mother, I hate you.

T. And then you tell her why you hate her.

C. You destroyed me.

T. That right. I hate you and you destroyed me. What you see, you made. You did it. It's your fault and you cannot plead ignorance. You should have known. You should have been better read. You should have been a better person. You shouldn't have made me so fearful of every little thing. And now I've killed hundreds of people. And it's your fault. Tell her that.

C. You . . .

T. (*Interrupting*) You see her face.

C. You didn't know that you were doing it, but you should have done a better job. Now you've made me crazy and I've killed hundreds of people.

T. That's right. And I hate you for it.

C. And I hate you for it.

T. Then she says, "I didn't mean to, I didn't know." And you say, "That's no excuse. That's no excuse for any mother to destroy her kid."

C. That's no excuse for any mother to destroy her kid.

T. You've destroyed me. Not only that, but you've made me miserable. Miserable, practically every day of my life I've been miserable. And I've suffered and it's all because of you. I want you to feel that now. Feel that it really is because of her. And it's her fault and she destroyed you. And you see her face and you say, "I hate you for it. I hate you for what you've done to me. I hate you. I hate you. And you goofed me up so much I've passed it on. And it's all your fault. For generation after generation you've passed this craziness down. It's your fault. You started it all." And you say, "I hate you. I hate you." See her and tell her that.

C. I hate you. I hate you. You've passed this on from generation to generation and I hate you for it.

T. That's right. And then you take your hand. And in a slow motion you see your hand and you see her face and you see your hand and you strike her across the face as hard as you can. You see that?

C. Um hum.

T. You see your hand coming out there and it hits her right across her face. And you hit her again and again and again and then you take your fist and you start hitting her. And you've got superhuman strength now, and you just start ripping her and hitting her and kicking her, kicking her, and you tear her hair out. You tear her hair out and you choke her. You choke her. And you kick her and you go crazy now. You go crazy. Your own mother, you take her and you pick her up and you slam her against the floor now. You slam her against the floor and you beat her about the head, again and again and again. You beat the rest of her body now. You punch her in the breasts. In her legs, in her arms, her neck, her eyes. And you just beat and kick her and then you start jumping up and down on her. She's on the floor now and you jump up and down on her and you say, "I hate you, I hate you, I hate you," everytime you jump, "I hate you, I hate you, I hate you." And you see yourself jumping and putting your heels into her. I hate you, I hate you. And you jump on her and you kill her. And jump on her and kill her and jump on her and kill her. Do you see that?

C. Yes.

T. See it. Again and again and again. She's down there. I hate you I hate you. Say that and jump on her.

C. I hate you. I hate you.

T Right. And you see her. And you feel that hate. I want you to really feel that hate. Because she really destroyed you. She really destroyed you! She made you crazy and you've suffered for it. And you know you'll suffer more for it now that you're crazy and you just jump on her—I hate you, I hate you, I hate you. You've really gone crazy now. You tell her that. Jump on her and tell her that. I hate you!

C. I hate you. I hate you.

T. That's right. Again.

C. I hate you.

T. OK. With some feeling now. You see her there.

C. I HATE you!

T. That's right. Tell her again the same way.
C. I HATE you!
T. Very good, again.
C. I HATE YOU!
T. Again.
C. I HATE YOU!
T. Again.
C I HATE YOU!
T. That's right. And you just hit her now. You hit her. You hit her. See yourself hitting her, again and again and again and again. (*Client sobbing*) You see yourself hitting her. Do you see that?
C. Um hum.
T. You're hitting her, again and again and again. And you just keep hitting her and hitting her and hitting her and hitting her and hitting her. And then you take her and you throw her against the wall. Right? You see that?
C. Um hum.
T. And then you pick her up and you throw her right out the window. Right out of the window. Her dead body now. You've killed her. You see that, you've killed her. A hundred and one people. And your mother. You've killed your mother. Do you see that?
C. Yes.
T. That's right. That's right. (*Client sobs*) And then somebody comes through the door. And you hear a male voice and he says, "What's going on here?" And you look around and it's your father. You see that?
C. Uh huh.
T. It's your father. And you say, "I hate you, too." You look at him and you say, "I hate you, too."
C. I hate you, too.
T. That's right. This is your natural father. You see that? The one that left you when you were four and helpless. At least, your mother tried; at least, she tried. She may have really goofed it up, in fact, she did, but she tried and you look at your father and you say, "At least, Mother tried."
C. At least, Mother tried.
T. That's right. And tell him, "You left me."
C. You left when I was four.
T. You didn't even care for me enough to visit.
C. You didn't even care enough to visit.
T. He makes some feeble excuse. He says, "I was busy. I was busy." And you say, "You shit. You shit. You are the lowest thing on this earth; who would leave his little boy helpless with a crazy mother and leave him, leave him to go crazy like I've gone crazy right now? You see me. I am crazy and I hate you and I am going to kill you." Tell him that.
C. I'm sorry, I messed up.
T. That's all right. You see his face there.
C. Uh huh.
T. You see his face there and you say, "You deserted me."

C. You deserted me.

T. And I hate you.

C. And I hate you and I'm going to kill you.

T. That's right. And tell him the same thing again. You see his face there. He looks kind of startled. And you tell him that.

C. You deserted me and I hate you and I'm going to kill you.

T. That's right. And you go over to him and you remember, it goes through your mind like it was happening right now, right today, you remember when you were a little boy. You remember that he deserted you and, in fact, you even have a memory of him beating on you before he left. Beating on you. He hated you. You can remember. It's clear as day. He hated you, a little helpless child. And he made you crazy. He made you crazy. You thought it was your mother, but he beat on you. He beat on you. And then he deserted you. And you feel that. No love. No love from him. Hate, hate and you go up and you start hitting him. You start hitting him. (*Client sobbing*) And you say, "I hate you, I hate you, I hate you." You see that?

C. Uh huh.

T. "I hate you." And you start beating on him. "You shit. You turd. You low nothing of a man. You deserve everything you get." And you give it to him. You start hitting him again and again and again and again. You hit him, beat him, scratch him, tear his hair out. You kick him in the genitals now. You kick him in the genitals and you destroy his genitals. You destroy his genitals. He's not a man. A man wouldn't beat on a little four-year-old. And you kick and you destroy his genitals. And then you stomp on him and kick him and jump up and down and you say, "I hate you, I hate you, I hate you for what you did to me. I hate you for what you've done to me. Look, Father, what you've done to your own son. Look, Father, what you've done to me." And you're crazy now. You're really crazy, and you jump up and down on him and you jump up and down on him. And you dig your heels in. You dig your heels into him. Yes, you see that. Now you feel his flesh beneath you. And you dig your heels into him and you say, "I hate you, I hate you, I hate you, I hate you, I hate you." And you just destroy him. Destroy him and you hit him again and again and again. Do you see that?

C. Um hum.

T. Then you lean over and you pick him up and you put him up against the wall and hit him some more. You hit him again and again and again. And everytime you see his face you remember what he did to you. You remember. He deserted you and you remember that. You can even remember he mistreated you and you're paying him back finally now, you're paying him back. And you hit him again and again and again. You see that?

C. Um hum.

T. Hit him. And say that everytime you hit him.

C. I hate you. I hate you, I hate you.

T. And then you kick him and do the same thing.

C. I hate you, I hate you, I hate you. (*As he kicks in the air*)

T. That's right. And then you pick him up. You pick him up and then you throw him on the floor. And you jump on him some more. You jump on him again and again and again and again. And you jump on him. Hate, hate, hate. And you rip him up. And you say, "You abused me. You didn't love me. You're a son-of-a-bitch." And you kill him. You kill him. You see that. Tell him that. "You're a son-of-a-bitch and you deserve to die," and you hit him again.

C. You're a son-of-a-bitch and you deserve to die.

T. That's right and you hit him again and again and again and again. You rip his body up. You just rip it up. You have superhuman strength. It's like he's a four-year-old and you're an adult now. And he's the dependent one. And you have him right where you want him. And you pay him back. You take him and you just rip him up now. You rip him up. You rip up his genitals, 'cause he's not a man. (*Client sobbing*) You rip up his genitals, that's right. You take his genitals and you grap his penis there and you just rip it off, that's right. You hook your fingerhails into it and you just rip it off. You rip it off, that's right. And you stomp on his testicles and squish them. You squish them and then you take your foot and you kick him right in the butt. You kick him there and you jump up and down on him some more. Jump up and down on him some more, and you're really crazy now. You're really crazy. You ripped his genitals off. And you smashed him and you hit his face. You start kicking his face now, and putting your heel into it. And you just kill him, smash him. Smash him. You see that?

C. Um hum.

T. You're crazy now. You smash him. Smash him. And finally you just say, "You've got yours now, what does it feel like?"

C. You've got yours now, what does it feel like?

T. And he doesn't say anything. He just lays there and he moans and you say, "You deserve it." Feel it. Feel it. "You deserve it. Suffer like I've suffered. You're lucky. You suffered for only five minutes, I suffered for years, decades, all of my life. And he lays there and moans. And you just watch him moan and then you kick him again. "Feel it," you say as you kick him. "Feel it. Feel it. I feel it. I still feel it." And you kick him and kick him and kick him and kick him and kick him and kick him and put your heel into him. And you find the place that makes him moan the most and you kick him there. You kick him there, and you say, "Feel it, Dad. Feel it. You deserve to suffer." And you just kill him. Kill him. And then you take his body and you throw it out the window in a heap. And he's dead now. He's dead. The life seeps out of him and you take his body and you throw it out in a heap. And then is there anybody else that comes through that door?

C. No.

T. No. Nobody else until the sirens come. And they come in and they've got white coats on. And they come in and you're just sitting there. You're just sitting there and your mind's a blank. Your mind's a blank. And you're just sitting there. You don't even resist. They take you and they strap you down. They strap you down. Feel that now. They strap you down and they take you to a very high security criminal mental institution. It's got bars. And bars and doors and steel doors and more bars. And they take you in and they strap you down. They strap you down. You feel that?

C. Um hum.

T. And they show you no mercy. No mercy. Everytime you say, "I'm hungry, I'm thirsty, I'm anxious, help me," they look down at you and they say, "You are a bad person. You've killed a hundred and two people. You killed your own parents. You killed a hundred therapists. You killed your mother and you killed your father and you deserve to suffer." And you try to tell them, "They made me suffer. They deserved it." And they just shake their heads. And they say, "You're crazy. You're really crazy. Crazy or not you deserve to suffer." You see that?

C. Um hum.

T. "Crazy or not you deserve to suffer," and they tell you that. And then, one of them comes, a particularly big fellow, and he looks down and he looks like he really knows a lot, and he gets this knowing look on his face and he looks down and he says, "You're crazy because you were a sinner, not because of your parents or your therapists or your Dad or your Mom, or anybody. Because you were a bad person. That's why you're crazy. This is your punishment. And you deserve it 'cause you're a bad person." Can you feel that?

C. Uh huh.

T. And you know he's right. I want you to feel that he's right. Can you feel that? He's really right. It wasn't your Mom or your Dad or any of those other people. It's you. And you are suffering because you deserve it and it starts running through your mind. Starts running through your mind about all the things you've done wrong. Which one is God punishing you for? And you try to think, even though your mind is hazy. It runs through your mind what you did. Your pettiness, sexual things when you were sixteen, you remember when you masturbated, that runs through your mind. And you feel dirty and guilty and you remember masturbating and you remember what you've done to your daughter. You remember that maybe your mother did wrong, but you knew and you just passed it along. You knowingly passed it along. And that passes through your mind. And you know that he's right. He's right. You really did wrong. And that's why you're suffering. That's why you're crazy. I want you to feel that. What else runs through your mind as he looks down at you and says, "You're suffering because you're guilty and you're a sinner?"

C. That he's right.

T. What kind of things run through your mind that you've done wrong in your lifetime.

C. The things you mentioned.

T. That's right. Anything else?

C. No.

T. You remember masturbating. And touching yourself down there, don't you?

C. Um hum.

T. That's right. And you know about the petting, you remember that. Letting her touch you. You did that. You weren't even married and you did that. You did it more than once, didn't you? And you remember it. And you knew it was wrong. You knew it was wrong. You didn't care. All you wanted was your own pleasure. That's all you wanted. You didn't care about God or what was right. And you know that you're suffering now because of that. And now you've killed your own parents. You killed your mother. You feel that? You killed her. She tried her best, and it wasn't her fault that she had a crazy son. That wasn't her fault. Then about your father, he left you and you started to wonder what kind of a terrible kid you were that you drove him out of the house. I want you to feel that now. What kind of a terrible kid were you that you made him leave? That's right, you must have done something pretty bad to drive him out. So bad that he couldn't stand you and he didn't even want to have contact with you. You drove him out and then you killed him. Brutally. You killed your mother who stuck by you all these years. You killed her, too. And you didn't kill your daughter, but you raised her around all your neurotic things, didn't you?

C. Yes.

T. And she looks pretty straight now, but you used to look pretty straight, too. What will happen when she gets a little older? What will happen? Will she go crazy? Just like this? What will happen? You used to be the big jock. You used to be into a lot of things. You didn't used to be that anxious. And then you went crazy. Didn't you? You went slowly crazy. Slowly crazy and they put you in a mental hospital and you killed people and you went crazy. What will happen to her? What will happen to her? Your own daughter, what have you done to her? That all goes through your mind. You see that? You see that?

C. Yes. (*Sobbing*)

T. That's right. You feel it now. You feel it. (*Client actively sobbing*) You're responsible. I want you to feel that now. You're really responsible. You feel that. (*More sobbing*) You feel that? What are you feeling right now, sad about your daughter?

C. Yes. (*Sobbing*)

T. That's right. That's right. You feel that. Like you've really ruined her life. Maybe it hasn't shown up yet, but you know it will. (*Client sobbing*) You know it will. That's right. You know it will show up. You know it will show up. (*Client sobbing*) You've ruined her life. You've ruined her life. And what did she ever do to you? Nothing. Nothing. The doctors let you sit there and suffer, but you don't complain any longer. You don't complain. You feel the pain of hunger and thirst and the bindings on your arms. And you hear yourself ranting and raving like it was another person. But you don't complain now because you know you deserve it. You know you deserve it. It was really your fault all along. Really your fault. Do you feel that?

C. Um hum.

T. And it runs through your mind about your daughter—what you did to your daughter. What did you do to her? What goes through your mind?

C. Like you said, that I was neurotic and it hasn't shown up yet, but . . . (*Breaks down sobbing*)

T. Maybe it will. And if it does, oh, you'll feel it's your fault. Really your fault. You used to think you tried your best, but maybe you didn't, you didn't do enough—

C. I guess I'm getting what I've done.

T. That's right. It starts to run through your mind. That justice has been done. You're really getting what you deserve. And you start to welcome the pain almost.

C. Yes.

T. You're getting what you deserve. You've sinned. And you just lay there and suffer and suffer and suffer the pain, the thirst, the hunger, and the degradation of having no place to go to the bathroom. Nobody to touch you or care about you. It just goes on and on and on and on. Nobody loves you, nobody loves you. Pay attention to your bodily sensations now; what do you feel in your body?

C. I'm just as tight as I can be all over.

T. All your muscles now; pay attention to them; they're all tight.

C. Yes.

T. They're all tight. Your arms, your legs, your bottom, your front, everything's tight.

C. Yes.

T. Your neck, forehead, everything. And you feel guilt. You still feel that guilt?

C. Yes.

T. You feel other emotions?

C. A fear, I guess.

T. What do you fear? What do you fear now?

C. I fear that, that maybe someday something will happen to Jenny and it will be my fault.

T. Someday she'll go crazy and have a rough time.

C. Oh. *(Pained)*

T. Is that what you feel?

C. Yes.

T. And she'll have to really suffer. And it'll be all your fault.

C. Yes.

T. Right now you're suffering. You're suffering. You're tied down to that—strapped down to that table. Strapped down to that table and you're hungry and cold and nobody loves you. Can you feel that?

C. Uh huh.

T. Nobody loves you. And they don't even feed you. They don't talk to you. They glower at you. Hate, that's all, that's all. And you feel like you deserve it. And they just hate you. And you're wrapped and tied and bound and hungry and cold and cold and hungry and thirsty. And you have your bowel movements right there on the table. They don't feed you. And you're a mess. You can't do any rituals or anything because you're strapped down and nobody loves you. You feel that?

C. Yes.

T. What thoughts are going through your mind?

C. I feel like . . . I can't do any rituals, but I can't do anything else either.

T. What else would you want to do?

C. Well, I don't want to be crazy. I just want to live normally and naturally . . .

T. You feel like there's a good part to being strapped down? At least, you can't do anything crazy?

C. No, I don't feel that way at all.

T. But you feel regret at being treated that way, not being allowed to move or do anything. Or talk to people. Maybe you could make up for what you've done, but they don't let you. They don't give you any more chances at all. They just leave you tied down and suffering. Do you feel that?

C. Um hum.

T. Tied down and suffering. And it just goes on and on and on. There's no let up. OK., you can open your eyes. You want to move around a little bit? Move your legs and your arms. How do you feel?

C. Terrible.

T. Terrible? . . . Are you out of the scene?

C. Oh yes, completely.

T. OK. Do you still feel real tense or tired or both?

C. Very tense.

T. More tense than tired?

C. Yes.

T. You seemed to get into that scene real well.

C. Yeah, I was there. I'm almost still there.

T. Are you stuck in the last part of it or are you still someplace else?

C. No, it's just, just the whole thing. Mostly the last part, I guess. My head is splitting. (*Pause*) You know this therapy is making me feel that I've lost control.

T. Um hum.

C. That I don't know what I'm doing. Is that good?

T. Well, I think it is. In other words, I think that ultimately you'll be happier if you can let go of some of the control. I think you hold onto more control than you really need, and it keeps you from being free and happy. You feel uptight and if you lose a little of that, for whatever reason, whether you decide to or you just have a hard time holding onto it, I think that ultimately you'll become comfortable with a little less control. And then maybe you can lose a little more and become comfortable with that, and so on.

C. Yeah, I agree with that, but I get into it so, and I'm so suggestible that I feel that I really have lost it.

T. Into the scene, you're talking about?

C. No.

T. What?

C. All the time.

T. Um hum. You get into your doubt so much that you . . .

C. (*Interrupting*) Uh huh.

T. But you haven't. You're here and you're sensible and that's what you'll slowly learn over time, that you can, in a sense, go crazy and then be uncrazy. It's not that you have control over it all the time. You don't have to watch it every second, like you do. You're always on guard.

C. Right.

T. And really most people don't, because they know it's normal to be crazy once in awhile, and they can always bring it back.

C. Yes.

T. And you at a real gut level, not up in your head, but at a real gut level, don't know that yet. And you have to learn it slowly, painfully sometimes.
C. Very painfully.
T. But I think the more deeply and completely you get into the scene the quicker you'll learn. And it may seem to you that, in effect, living the kind of thing that you fear, that's the most painful thing for anybody to do.
C. Yes.
T. Emotionally painful, if not physically.
C. Um hum.
T. But I think that's it's good.
C. Well, I really get into it.
T. Well, this one you did, very much. How would you rate it?
C. I'd rate that 100!
T. 100 or 110, huh?
C. Yeah, that's about right, 500.
T. OK. I want to talk to you about changing your eating ritual so it's less logical.
C. Right.
T. You said that you normally drink your tea before dessert. That one thing you could do is drink some tea after dessert.
C. Um hum.
T. You don't have dessert with every meal, do you?
C. Yeah.
T. Really? Breakfast?
C. Oh no, not breakfast. I don't eat breakfast.
T. Oh.
C. But I do with lunch and dinner.
T. Why don't you eat breakfast?
C. I just never have.
T. I guess I'm still kind of curious about your being more shaky in the morning.
C. Uh huh. Well, maybe that would help.
T. I wonder. I don't know, but I know if I don't eat breakfast, particularly some protein like milk or something that has protein in it, I am shaky until I eat, and you did say that you feel better after lunch.
C. Yeah, it could be that.
T. Try drinking some milk or something. What else could you change about your eating ritual? You said you had to put the utensil on the last plate that it's been used on. It's sort of the utensil that's appropriate to the food then.
C. Right.
T. Could you put the utensils on inappropriate plates? You know what I mean? Put your spoon on the table and put your knife where the cake was, rather than the fork, or something like that. More or less rearrange them. Do you think you could carry that out? How much anxiety would you experience upon doing that or after doing that?
C. Well, some but, if it would help, I'll try it.
T. OK. There is another thing I'd like you to start trying. You say you're having more doubt during the day about whether you've done something this way or that way or another way. And you have trouble remembering it. What

I'd like you to do at those times, when you normally would close your eyes and try to get it straight, I'd like you to try closing your eyes and increasing your doubt. That's what we did here when you were—

C. (*Interrupting*) That's going to be really hard.

T. Uh huh, OK. Can you live with the doubt and try to lessen the number of times you stop and think about it?

C. I can try that.

T. I actually think you've done that already. But I'm not sure you'd agree.

C. Yeah, I think maybe I have.

T. At least, you no longer stop me or want me to repeat things or have to wait a minute to go over what I've said; whereas before, you used to do that quite a bit. And Dr. Smith reports that he thinks that's true on the ward, too. You have to pause less often. If you think that doing a little scary scene would be too much for you at this point in the therapy, you could, instead, try increasing the number of times that you don't think of it and you just kind of stay with the doubt as long as you can.

C. OK.

T. I'd like you to get to the point where you could live with doubt without it being a big thing.

C. Yes, I understand that's the reason for it.

T. Also, I'd like you to do the scene we did today a couple of times a day. OK. Do you remember it?

C. Yes.

T. I'm not sure I do; that's why I asked. Starting with the cigarette, I guess, and progressing to going crazy and for awhile . . .

C. (*Interrupting*) . . . and killing everyone on the ward.

T. Going crazy will mean being hostile and first you confront a lot of different people and you express anger verbally. In your mind, or if nobody's around you can say it out loud. And then physically by hitting them, and then by killing them. OK.? Including important people on the ward, myself, Dr. Smith and people in your life outside of the ward. And then the rest of it as you've been pretty much doing already, OK.?

Steve was discharged from the hospital after ten implosive therapy sessions (over a six-week period). His pretherapy MMPI profile was markedly elevated (278* 60′) and suggestive of subjective distress, obsessive ideation, fears of loss of control, suspiciousness, and social withdrawal. The post therapy MMPI profile showed great improvement with only the subjective distress scales somewhat elevated (27′). The number and duration of compulsive rituals was reduced. Steve was able, for example, to complete his morning routine in less than an hour (down from three hours). His fear of expressing anger was greatly reduced; he was, for example, able to express appropriate anger toward his parents. And he was making plans to move from his parents home to live independently. The fear of losing control and going crazy was still present to some degree. He occasionally attempted to recall and recreate things in his mind, and still had an overconcern with whether his cigarette was put out "properly."

EPILOGUE

We set out to (1) dispel the notion that exposure therapies are dangerous or harmful or have more negative side effects than other therapies, and (2) teach others how to use these techniques that we have found so effective with our clients over the years. We have presented evidence that direct therapeutic exposure is especially effective for certain anxiety-based disorders, and in fact may be the treatment of choice for phobics and obsessive-compulsive clients. The unfounded concerns about the dangers of these techniques have, in effect, resulted in clients receiving less effective treatment than might otherwise have been given. This is especially unfortunate for the mental health professions where highly efficient and effective treatments are not easy to come by.

In 1967, in one of the episodes of the interesting and compelling television series, *The Twenty-First Century,* CBS televised Thomas Stampfl and Donald Levis, using implosive therapy with a young phobic secretary. At that time, there was little evidence for the effectiveness of implosive therapy or the flooding technique. The narrator, Walter Cronkite, described Stampfl as a "far-out member of a school of therapists called Behaviorists." But he also noted that regardless of how the therapy looks to the layman, it was a good bet that by the twenty-first century there would be more "tension, more stress, more fear" around, and that the only criterion for determining which therapy to use would be "what works." It is not the twenty-first century yet, but the data are in. Therapeutic exposure not only works, but it is safe and efficient. Far-out is now in, and we had better use these techniques if we want to give our clients effective treatment.

REFERENCES

Adams, H. E., & Hughes, H. H. Animals analogues of behavioral treatment procedures: A critical evaluation. In M. Herson, R. M. Eisler, & P. M. Miller (Eds.), *Progress in behavior modification* (Vol. 2). New York: Academic Press, 1976.

Adams, H. E., & Hughes, H. H. Animal analogues of behavioral treatment procedures: A critical evaluation. In M. Herson, R. M. Eisler, & P. M. Miller (Eds.), *Progress in behavior modification* (Vol. 3). New York: Academic Press, 1976.

Antman, E. Flooding *in vivo* for a case of vermiphobia. *Journal of Behavior Therapy and Experimental Psychology*, 1973, 4, 275–277.

Ayer, W. A. Implosive therapy: A review. *Psychotherapy: Theory, Research and Practice*, 1972, *9*, 242–250.

Bandura, A. *Principles of behavior modification.* New York: Holt, Rinehart & Winston, 1969.

Bandura, A. On paradigms and recycled ideologies. *Cognitive Theory and Research*, 1978, *2*, 79–103.

Bankart, B., & Elliott, R. Extinction of avoidance in rats: Response availability and stimulus presentation effects. *Behaviour Research and Therapy*, 1974, *12*, 53–56.

Barlow, D. H., & Wolfe, B. E. Behavioral approaches to anxiety disorders: A report on the NIMH-SUNY Albany research conference. *Journal of Consulting and Clinical Psychology*, 1981, *49*, 448–455.

Barrios, B. A. Publication trends in behavior therapy analogue research on phobias. *Journal of Behavior Therapy and Experimental Psychiatry*, 1979, *10*, 203–205.

Baum, M. Rapid extinction of an avoidance response following a period of response prevention in the avoidance apparatus. *Psychological Report*, 1966, *18*, 59–64.

Baum, M. Extinction of an avoidance response motivated by intense fear: Social facilitation of the action of response prevention (flooding) in rats. *Behaviour Research and Therapy*, 1969, *7*, 57–62.

Baum, M. Extinction of avoidance responding through response prevention (flooding). *Psychological Bulletin*, 1970, *77*, 276–284.

Baum, M. Extinction of avoidance in rats: The effects of chlorpromazine and methylphenidate administered in conjunction with flooding (response prevention). *Behavior Research and Therapy*, 1973, *11*, 165–169.

Baum, M., & Gordon, A. Effects of a loud buzzer applied during response prevention (flooding) in rats. *Behaviour Research and Therapy*, 1970, *8*, 287–292.

Baum, M., & LeClerc, R. Irrelevant stress versus response prevention (flooding) interpolated between avoidance acquisition and extinction in rats. *Journal of Psychiatric Research*, 1974, *10*, 307–314.

Baum, M., & Poser, E. G. Comparison of flooding procedures in animals and man. *Behaviour Research and Therapy*, 1971, *9*, 249–254.

Berger, L., & McGaugh, J. L. Critique and reformulation of "Learning Theory" approaches to psychotherapy and neurosis. *Psychological Bulletin*, 1965, *63*, 338–358.

Berman, J. S., & Katzev, R. D. Factors involved in the rapid elimination of avoidance behavior. *Behaviour Research and Therapy*, 1972, *10*, 247–256.

Bernstein, D. A. Behavioral fear assessment: Anxiety or artifact? In H. Adams & I. P. Unilcel (Eds.), *Issues and trends in behavior therapy*. Springfield, Ill.: Charles C Thomas, 1973.

Bernstein, D. A., & Borkovec, T. D. *Progressive relaxation training: A manual for the helping professions*. Champaign, Ill.: Research Press, 1973.

Bernstein, D. A., & Nietzel, M. T. Demand characteristics in behavior modification: The natural history of a "nuisance". In M. Hersen, R. M. E. Eisler, & P. Miller (Eds.), *Progress in behavior modification*, New York: Academic Press, 1977.

Bersh, P. J., & Keltz, J. R. Avoidance behavior in rats after extinction with response prevention. *Journal of Comparative and Physiological Psychology*, 1971, *76*, 262–266.

Bersh, P. J., & Miller, K. The influence of shock during response prevention upon resistance to extinction of an avoidance response. *Animal Learning and Behavior*, 1975, *3*, 140–142.

Bersh, P. J., & Paynter, W. E. Pavlovian extinction in rats during avoidance response prevention. *Journal of Comparative and Physiological Psychology*, 1972, *78*, 255–259.

Beutler, L. E. A self-directed approach to the treatment of a complex neurosis with implosive therapy. *Journal of Clinical Psychology*, 1973, *29*, 106–108.

Bijou, S. W. A conditioned response technique to investigate "experimental neurosis" in the rat. *Journal of Comparative and Physiological Psychology*, 1951, *44*, 84–87.

Black, A. H. The extinction of avoidance responses under Curare. *Journal of Comparative and Physiological Psychology*, 1958, *51*, 519–525.

Boersma, K., den Hengst, S., Dekker, J., & Emmelkamp, P.M.G. Exposure and response prevention in the natural environment: A comparison with obsessive-compulsive patients. *Behaviour Research and Therapy*, 1976, *14*, 19–24.

Borkovec, T. D. Effects of expectancy on the outcome of systematic desensitization and implosive treatments for analogue anxiety. *Behavior Therapy*, 1972, *3*, 29–40.

Borkovec, T. D. The role of expectancy and physiological feedback in fear research: A review with special reference to subject characteristics. *Behavior Therapy*, 1973, *4*, 491–505.

Borkovec, T. D. Heart-rate process during systematic desensitization and implosive therapy for analogue anxiety. *Behavior Therapy*, 1974, *5*, 636–641.

Borkovec, T. D., & Nau, S. D. Credibility of analogue therapy rationales. *Journal of Behavior Therapy and Experimental Psychiatry*, 1972, *3*, 257–260.

Borkovec, T. D., & O'Brien, G. T. Methodological and target behavior issues in analogue therapy outcome research. In M. Herson, R. M. Eisler, & P. M. Miller (Eds.), *Progress in behavior modification* (Vol. 3). New York: Academic Press, 1976.

Borkovec, T. D., & Rachman, S. The utility of analogue research. *Behaviour Research and Therapy*, 1979, *17*, 253–261.

Borkovec, T. D., & Sides, J. K. The contribution of relaxation and expectancy to fear reduction via graded imaginal exposure to feared stimuli. *Behaviour Research and Therapy*, 1979, *12*, 529–540.

Boudewyns, P. A. Is "milieu therapy" in a short-term inpatient psychiatric setting worth the money? *International Mental Health Research Newsletter*, 1974, *16*, 7–8.

Boudewyns, P. A. Implosive therapy and desensitization therapy with inpatients: A five-year followup. *Journal of Abnormal Psychology*, 1975, *84*, 159–160.

Boudewyns, P. A., & Borkovec, T. D. Credibility of psychotherapy and placebo therapy rationales. *V. A. Newsletter for Research in Mental Health and Behavioral Sciences*, 1974, *16*, 15–18.

Boudewyns, P. A., & Levis, D. J. Autonomic reactivity of high and low ego-strength subjects to repeated anxiety-eliciting scenes. *Journal of Abnormal Psychology*, 1975, *84*, 682–692.

Boudewyns, P. A., & Shipley, R. Confusing negative practice with flooding: A cautionary note. *The Behavior Therapist*, 1982, *5*, 47–48.

Boudewyns, P. A., & Wilson, A. E. Implosive therapy and desensitization therapy using free association in treatment of inpatients. *Journal of Abnormal Psychology*, 1972, *79*, 259–268.

Boulougouris, J. C., Marks, I. M., & Marset, P. Superiority of flooding (implosion) to desensitization for reducing pathological fear. *Behaviour Research and Therapy*, 1971, *9*, 7–19.

Boulougouris, J. C., Rabavilas, A. D., & Stefanis, C. Physiological responses in obsessive-compulsive patients. *Behaviour Research and Therapy*, 1977, *15*, 221–230.

Boyd, T. L., & Levis, D. J. The effects of single-component extinction to a three-component serial CS on resistance to extinction of the conditioned avoidance response. *Learning and Motivation*, 1976, *7*, 517–531.

Broadhurst, P. L. Abnormal animal behavior. In H. J. Eysenck, (Ed.), *Handbook of abnormal psychology*. London: Pitman Medical Publishers, 1960.

Brown, J. S., & Jacobs, A. The role of fear in the motivation and acquisition of responses. *Journal of Experimental Psychology*, 1949, *39*, 747–759.

Brush, F. R. The effects of shock intensity on the acquisition and extinction of an avoidance response in dogs. *Journal of Comparative and Physiological Psychology*, 1957, *50*, 547–552.

Butollo, W., & Mittalstaedt, L. Systematic combination of treatment components: Self-instructional training, modeling with participation, post-treatment care in the behavioral modification of severe phobic disorders. In J. C. Boulougouris & A. D. Rabavilas (Eds.), *The treatment of phobic and obsessive-compulsive disorders*. Oxford: Pergamon, 1977

Campbell, D. T., & Stanley, J. C. *Experimental and quasi-experimental designs for research*. Chicago: Rand McNally, 1966.

Carlson, N. J., & Black, A. H. Traumatic avoidance learning: Note on the effect of response prevention during extinction. *Psychological Reports*, 959, *4*, 409–412.

Carrera, R. N., & Elenewski, J. J. Implosive therapy as a treatment for insomnia. *Journal of Clinical Psychology*, 1980, *36*, 729–734.

Cautela, J., & Baron, M. Covert conditioning: A theoretical analysis. *Behavior Modification*, 1977, *1*, 351–368.

Chambless, D. L., Foa, E. B., Groves, G. A., & Goldstein, A. J. Flooding with brevital in the treatment of agoraphobia. *Behaviour Research and Therapy*, 1979, *17*, 243–251.

Chambless, D. L., Foa, E. B., Groves, G. A., & Goldstein, A. J. *The role of anxiety in flooding with agoraphobics*. Paper presented at the meeting of the American Psychological Association, Montreal, September 1980.

Chambless, D. L., & Goldstein, A. J. Clinical treatment of agoraphobia. In M. Mavissakalian & D. H. Barlow (Eds.), *Phobia*. New York: Guilford Press, 1981.

Chaplin, E. W., & Levine, B. A. The effects of total exposure duration and interrupted versus continuous exposure in flooding therapy. *Behavior Therapy*, 1981, *12*, 360–368.

Christy, D., & Reid, L. Methods of deconditioning persisting avoidance: Amphetamine, and amobarbital as adjuncts to response prevention. *Bulletin of Psychonomic Society*, 1975, *5*, 175–177.

Coleman, J. C. *Abnormal psychology and modern life.* (5th ed.) Glenview, Ill.: Scott, Foresman, 1976.

Cook, S. W. A survey of methods used to produce "experimental neurosis." *American Journal of Psychiatry,* 1939, *95,* 259–276.

Cooper, S., Coon, K., Mejta, C., & Reid, L. Methods of deconditioning persisting avoidance: Amphetamine, chlorpromazine, and chlordiazepoxide as adjuncts to response prevention. *Physiological Psychology,* 1974, *3,* 519–522.

Cooper, A., Furst, J. B., & Bridger, W. G. A brief commentary on the usefulness of studying fears of snakes. *Journal of Abnormal Psychology,* 1969, *74,* 408–414.

Corriveau, D. P., & Smith, N. F. Fear reduction and "safety-test" behavior following response prevention: A multivariate analysis. *Journal of Experimental Psychology,* 1978, *107,* 145–158.

Coulter, X., Riccio, D. C., & Page, H. A. Effects of blocking an instrumental avoidance response: Facilitated extinction but persistence of "fear." *Journal of Comparative and Physiological Psychiatry,* 1969, *68,* 377–381.

Crowe, M. J., Marks, I. M., Agras, W. S., & Leitenberg, H. Time-limited desensitization, implosion and shaping for phobic patients: A crossover study. *Behaviour Research and Therapy,* 1972, *10,* 319–328.

Denholtz, W. The use of tape recordings during therapy sessions. *Journal of Behavior Therapy and Experimental Psychiatry,* 1970, *1,* 139–143.

Dollard, J., & Miller, N. E. *Personality and psychotherapy.* New York: McGraw-Hill, 1950.

Drummond, P., White, K., & Ashton, R. Imagery vividness affects habituation rate. *Psychophysiology,* 1978, *15,* 193–195.

Edinger, J. D., & Jacobson, R. Incidence and significance of relaxation treatment side effects. *The Behavior Therapist,* 1982, *5,* 137–138.

Ellis, A. *Reason and emotion in psychotherapy.* New York: Lyle Stuart, 1962.

Emmelkamp, P. M. G. Self observation vs. flooding in the treatment of agoraphobia. *Behaviour Research and Therapy,* 1974, *12,* 229–237.

Emmelkamp, P. M. G., & Kraanen, J. Therapist-controlled exposure *in vivo* versus self-controlled exposure *in vivo*: A comparison with obsessive-compulsive patients. *Behaviour Research and Therapy,* 1977, *15,* 491–495.

Emmelkamp, P. M. G., Kuipers, A. C. M., & Eggeraat, J. B. Cognitive modification versus prolonged exposure *in vivo*: A comparison with agoraphobics as subjects. *Behaviour Research and Therapy,* 1978, *16,* 33–41.

Emmelkamp, P. M. G., & Kwee, K. G. Obsessional ruminations: A comparison between thought-stopping and prolonged exposure in imagination. *Behaviour Research and Therapy,* 1977, *15,* 441–444.

Emmelkamp, P. M. G., & Ultee, K. A. A comparison of "successive approximation" and "self-observation" in the treatment of agoraphobia. *Behavior Therapy,* 1974, *5,* 606–613.

Emmelkamp, P. M. G., & Wessels, H. Flooding in imagination vs. flooding *in vivo*: A comparison with agoraphobics. *Behaviour Research and Therapy,* 1975, *13,* 7–15.

Everaerd, W. T. A. M., Rijken, H. M., & Emmelkamp, P. M. G. A comparison of "flooding" and "successive approximation" in the treatment of agoraphobia. *Behaviour Research and Therapy,* 1973, *11,* 105–117.

Eysenck, H. J. A theory of the incubation of anxiety/fear responses. *Behaviour Research and Therapy,* 1968, *6,* 390–322.

Fairbank, J. A., & Keane, T. M. *Flooding for combat-related stress disorder: Assessment of anxiety reduction across traumatic memories.* Paper presented at the meeting of the Association for Advancement of Behavior Therapy. Toronto, November 1981.

Fazio, A. F. Treatment components in implosive therapy. *Journal of Abnormal Psychology,* 1970, *76,* 211–219.

Fenichel, O. *The psychoanalytic theory of neurosis.* New York: Norton, 1945.

Foa, E. B., & Chambless, D. L. Habituation of subjective anxiety during flooding in imagery. *Behaviour Research and Therapy,* 1978, *16,* 391–399.

Foa, E. B., Blau, J., Prout, M., & Latimer, P. Is "horror" a necessary component of flooding (implosion)? *Behaviour Research and Therapy,* 1977, *15,* 397–402.

Foa, E. B., & Goldstein, A. A continuous exposure and complete response presentation in the treatment of obsessive compulsive neurosis. *Behavior Therapy,* 1978, *9,* 821–829.

Foa, E. B., & Steketee, G. S. Obsessive-compulsives: Conceptual issues and treatment interventions. *Progress in Behavior Modification,* 1979, *8,* 1–53.

Foa, E. B., Steketee, G., Turner, R. M., & Fischer, S. C. Effects of imaginal exposure to feared disasters in obsessive-compulsive checkers. *Behaviour Research and Therapy,* 1980, *18,* 449–455.

Ford, D. H., & Urban, H. B. Psychotherapy, In P. R. Farnsworth (Ed.), *Annual Review of Psychology,* 1967, *18,* 333–372.

Franchina, J. J., Hauser, P. J., & Agee, C. M. Persistence of response prevention effects following retraining of escape behavior. *Behaviour Research and Therapy,* 1975, *13,* 1–6.

Frankel. A. Treatment of a multisymptomatic phobic by a self-directed, self-reinforced imagery technique: A case study. *Journal of Abnormal Psychology,* 1970, *76,* 496–499.

Frankel, A. Implosive therapy: A review. *Psychotherapy: Theory, Research, and Practice,* 1972, *9,* 251–255.

Freud, S., & Breuer, J. On the physical mechanism of hysterical phenomenon. In J. Riviere (Translator), *Collected papers* (Vol. 1). London: Hogarth Press, 1953. (Originally published, 1893.)

Gauthier, J., & Marshall, W. L. The determination of optimal exposure to phobic stimuli in flooding therapy. *Behaviour Research and Therapy,* 1977, *15,* 403–410.

Gelder, M. G., Bancroft, J. H. J., Gath, D. H., Johnston, D. W., Mathews, A. M., & Shaw, P. M. Specific and non-specific factors in behavior therapy. *British Journal of Psychiatry,* 1973, *123,* 445–462.

Ghose, L., Giddon, D., Shiere, F., & Eogels, L. Evaluation of sibling support. *Journal of Dentistry for Children,* 1969, *36,* 35–49.

Goethe, J. W. von. [Poetry and truth from my own life.] In R. O. Mood (Translator), *Goethe's autobiography.* Washington, D. C.: Public Affairs Press, 1949. (Originally published, 1770.)

Goldstein, A. J., & Chambless, D. L. A reanalysis of agoraphobia. *Behavior Therapy,* 1978, *9,* 47–59.

Goldstein, A. J. Psychotherapy research by extrapolation from social psychology. In A. P. Goldstein & S. J. Dean (Eds.), *The investigation of psychotherapy: Commentaries and readings.* New York: Wiley, 1966.

Gordon, R. An investigation into some of the factors that favour the formation of stereotyped images. *British Journal of Psychology,* 1949, *39,* 156–157.

Gordon, W. C., Smith, G. J., & Katz, D. S. Dual effects of response blocking following avoidance learning. *Behaviour Research and Therapy,* 1979, *17,* 479–487.

Griest, J., Marks, I. M., Berlin, F., Gournay, K., & Noshirvani, H. Avoidance versus confrontation of fear. *Behavior Therapy,* 1980, *11,* 1–14.

Grinker, R. R., & Spiegel, J. P. *Men under stress.* Philadelphia: Blackston, 1945.

Hafner, J. Catharsis during prolonged exposure for snake phobia: An agent of change? *American Journal of Psychiatry,* 1978, *135,* 247–248.

Hafner, J., & Marks, I. Exposure *in vivo* of agoraphobics: Contributions of diazepam, group exposure, and anxiety evocation. *Psychological Medicine,* 1976, *6,* 71–88.

Hall, J. C. Some conditions of anxiety extinction. *Journal of Abnormal and Social Psychology*, 1955, *51*, 126–132.

Hand, I., Lamontagne, Y., & Marks, I. M. Group exposure (flooding) *in vivo* for agoraphobics. *British Journal of Psychiatry*, 1974, *124*, 588–602.

Haney, J. N., & Euse, F. J. Skin conductance and heart rate response to neutral, positive, and negative imagery: Implications for covert behavior therapy procedures. *Behavior Therapy*, 1976, *7*, 494–503.

Hannie, T. J., & Adams, H. E. Modification of agitation by flooding: A preliminary study. *Journal of Behavior Therapy and Experimental Psychiatry*, 1974, *5*, 161–166.

Hirt, M., & Greenfield, H. Implosive therapy treatment of heroin addicts during methadone detoxification. *Journal of Consulting and Clinical Psychology*, 1979, *47*, 982–983.

Hiscock, M. Imagery assessment through self-report: What do imagery questions measure? *Journal of Consulting and Clinical Psychology*, 1978, *46*, 223–230.

Hodgson, R., Rachman, S., & Marks, I. M. The treatment of chronic obsessive-compulsive neurosis, followup and further findings. *Behaviour Research and Therapy*, 1972, *10*, 181–189.

Hogan, R. A. Implosive therapy in the short term treatment of psychotics. *Psychotherapy: Theory, Research, and Practice*, 1966, *3*, 25–31.

Hogan, R. A. The implosive technique. *Behaviour Research and Therapy*, 1968, *6*, 423–431.

Hughes, H., Holder, B., & Dubois, K. E. One session of flooding as treatment for conditioned avoidance responding in humans: Effects of individualization of treatment duration. *Psychological Reports*, 1978, *42*, 663–672.

Hull, C. L. *Principles of behavior*. New York: Appleton-Century-Crofts, 1943.

Hunt, H. F. Problems in the interpretation of "experimental neurosis." *Psychological Reports*, 1964, *15*, 27–35.

Hunt, H. F., & Brady, J. V. Some effects of punishment and intercurrent "anxiety" on a simple operant. *Journal of Comparative and Physiological Psychology*, 1955, *48*, 305–310.

Hussain, M. Z. Desensitization and flooding (implosion) in treatment of phobias. *American Journal of Psychiatry*, 1971, *127*, 1509–1514.

Johnston, D., & Gath, D. Arousal level and attribution effects in diazepam-assisted flooding. *British Journal of Psychiatry*, 1973, *123*, 463–466.

Johnston, D. W., Lancashire, M., Mathews, A. M., Munby, M., Shaw, P. M., & Gelder, M. G. Imaginal flooding and exposure to real phobic situations: Changes during treatment. *British Journal of Psychiatry*, 1976, *129*, 372–377.

Kalish, H. I. Strength of fear as a function of the number of acquisition and extinction trials. *Journal of Experimental Psychology*, 1954, *47*, 1–9.

Kaloupek, D. G. The safety of an extinction approach to decreasing human fear: Examination of the incubation effect. In T. M. Keane (Chair), *Implosive (flooding) therapy: Theoretical advances and clinical application*. Symposium presented at the meeting of the Association for Advancement of Behavior Therapy, New York, November 1980.

Kamano, D. K. Joint effect of amobarbital and response prevention on avoidance extinction. *Psychological Report*, 1968, *22*, 544–546.

Kamano, D. K. Using drugs to modify the effect of response prevention on avoidance extinction. *Behaviour Research and Therapy*, 1972, *10*, 367–370.

Kamin, L. J., Brimer, C. J., & Black, A. H. Conditioned suppression as a monitor of fear of the CS in the course of avoidance training. *Journal of Comparative and Physiological Psychology*, 1963, *56*, 497–501.

Kandel, H. J., Ayllon, T., & Rosenbaum, M. S. Flooding or systematic exposure in the treatment of extreme social withdrawal in children. *Journal of Behavior Therapy and Experimental Psychiatry*, 1977, *8*, 75–81.

Kazdin, A. E. Evaluating the generality of findings in analogue therapy research. *Journal of Consulting and Clinical Psychology*, 1978, *46*, 673–686.

Keane, T. M., & Kaloupek, D. G. Imaginal flooding in the treatment of a post-traumatic stress disorder. *Journal of Consulting and Clinical Psychology*, 1982, *50*, 138–140.

Kimble, G. A. *Hilgard and Marquis' conditioning and learning*. New York: Appleton, 1961.

Kimble, G. A., & Kendall, J. W. A comparison of two methods of producing experimental extincton. *Journal of Experimental Psychology*, 1953, *45*, 87–90.

Lane, B. R., *The reduction of anxiety under three experimental conditions*. Unpublished doctoral dissertation, Columbia University, 1954.

Lang, P. J. Imagery in therapy: An information processing analysis of fear. *Behavior Therapy*, 1977, *8*, 862–886.

Lang, P. J., Melamed, B. G., & Hart, J. A. A physiological analysis of fear modification using an automated desensitization procedure. *Journal of Abnormal Psychology*, 1970, *76*, 230–234.

Lazarus, A. H. *Behavior therapy and beyond*. New York: McGraw-Hill, 1971.

Lederhendler, I., & Baum, M. Mechanical facilitation of the action of response prevention (flooding) in rats. *Behaviour Research and Therapy*, 1970, *8*, 43–48.

Levis, D. J. Implosive therapy, part III: The subhuman analogue, the strategy, and the technique. In S. G. Armitage (Ed.), *Behavorial modification techniques in the treatment of emotional disorders*. Battle Creek, Mich.: VA Publication, 1966, 22–37.

Levis, D. J. The case for performing research on nonpatient populations with fear of small animals: A reply to Cooper, Furst, and Bridger. *Journal of Abnormal Psychology*, 1970, *76* 36–38.

Levis, D. J., & Carrera, R. Effects of ten hours of implosive therapy in the treatment of outpatients: A preliminary report. *Journal of Abnormal Psychology*, 1967, *72*, 504–508.

Levis, D. J. & Hare, N. A review of the theoretical rationale and empirical support for the extinction approach of implosive (flooding) therapy. In M. Herson, R. M. Eisler, & P. M. Miller (Eds.), *Progress in behavior modification* (Vol. 4). New York: Academic Press, 1977.

Levis, D. J., & Stampfl, T. G. Effects of serial CS presentation on shuttlebox avoidance responding. *Learning and Motivation*, 1972, *3*, 73–90.

Lieb, J., Lipsitch, I. I., & Slaby, A. E. *The crisis team*. New York: Harper & Row, 1973.

Linton, J., Riccio, D., Rohrbaugh, M., & Page, H. The effects of blocking an instrumental avoidance response: Fear reduction or enhancement? *Behaviour Research and Therapy*, 1970, *8*, 267–272.

Lomont, J. F. Reciprocal inhibition or extinction? *Behaviour Research and Therapy*, 1965, *3*, 209–219.

London, P., *The modes and morals of psychotherapy*. New York: Holt, Rinehart & Winston, 1964.

Maier, N. R. F. *Studies of abnormal behavior in the rat: The neurotic pattern and an analysis of the situation which produces it*. New York: Harper, 1939.

Marks, I. M. Behavioral treatments of phobic and obsessive-compulsive disorders: A critical appraisal. In M. Hersen, R. M. Eisler, & P. M. Miller (Eds.), *Progress in behavior modification* (Vol. 1). New York: Academic Press, 1975.

Marks, I. M., Viswanathan, R., Lipsedge, M. S., & Gardner, R. Enhanced relief of phobias by flooding during waning diazepam effect. *British Journal of Psychiatry*, 1972, *121*, 493–505.

Marrazo, M. J., Riccio, D. C., & Riley, J. Effects of Pavlovian conditioned stimulus-unconditioned stimulus pairings during avoidance response-prevention trials in rats. *Journal of Comparative and Physiological Psychology*, 1974, *86*, 96–100.

Marshall, W. L., Gauthier, J., & Gordon, A. The current status of flooding therapy. In M. Hersen, R. Eisler, & P. Miller (Eds.), *Progress in behavior therapy*, 1979, *7*, 206–275.

Marzillier, J. S., Carroll, D., & Newland, J. R. Self-report and physiological changes accompanying repeated imagining of a phobic scene. *Behaviour Research and Therapy,* 1979, *17,* 71–77.

Mathews, A. M., Johnston, D., Lancashire, M., Munby, M., Shaw, P. M., & Gelder, M. G. Imaginal flooding and exposure to real phobic situation, treatment outcome with agoraphobic patients. *British Journal of Psychiatry,* 1976, *129,* 362–371.

Mathews, A. M., Johnston, D. W., Shaw, P. M., & Gelder, M. G. Process variables and the prediction of outcome in behaviour therapy. *British Journal of Psychiatry,* 1974, *125,* 256–264.

Mathews, A. M., & Shaw, P. Emotional arousal and persuasion effects in flooding. *Behaviour Research and Therapy,* 1973, *11,* 587–598.

Matthews, A., Teasdale, J., Munby, M., Johnston, D., & Shaw, P. A home-based treatment program for agoraphobia. *Behavior Therapy,* 1977, *8,* 915–924.

May, J. R. Psychophysiology of self-regulated phobic thoughts. *Behavior Therapy,* 1977, *8,* 150–159. (a)

May, J. R. A psychophysiological study of self and externally regulated phobic thought. *Behavior therapy,* 1977, *8,* 849–861. (b)

McAllister, W. R., & McAllister, D. E. Behavioral measurement of conditioned fear. In R. Brush (Ed.), *Aversive conditioning and learning.* New York: Academic Press, 1971.

McCarthy, B. W. Short-term implosive therapy: Case study. *Psychological Reports,* 1972, *30,* 589–590.

McCutcheon, B. A., & Adams, H. E. The physiological basis of implosive therapy. *Behaviour Research and Therapy,* 1975, *13,* 93–100.

McGlynn, F., & McDonnell, R. Subjective ratings of credibility following brief exposure to desensitization and pseudotherapy. *Behaviour Research and Therapy,* 1974, *12,* 141–146.

McLemore, C. W. Imagery in desensitization. *Behaviour Research and Therapy,* 1972, *10,* 52–57.

Miller, B. C., & Levis, D. J. The effects of varying short visual exposure times to a phobic test stimulus on subsequent avoidance behavior. *Behaviour Research and Therapy,* 1971, *9,* 17–21.

Mineka, S. The effects of flooding an irrelevant response in the extinction of avoidance responses. *Journal of Experimental Psychology: Animal Behavior Processes,* 1976, *2,* 142–153.

Mineka, S. The role of fear in theories of avoidance learning, flooding, and extinction. *Psychological Bulletin,* 1979, *86,* 985–1010.

Monti, P. M., & Smith, N. F. Residual fear of the conditioned stimulus as a function of response prevention after avoidance or classical defensive conditioning in the rat. *Journal of Experimental Psychology: General,* 1976, *105,* 148–162.

Morganstern, K. P. Implosive therapy and flooding procedures: A critical review. *Psychological Bulletin,* 1973, *79,* 318–334.

Morokoff P. J., & Timberlake, W. Cue exposure and overt fear responses as determinants of extinction of avoidance in rats. *Journal of Comparative and Physiological Psychology,* 1971, *77,* 432–438.

Mowrer, O. H. On the dual nature of learning—a reinterpretation of "conditioning" and "problem-solving." *Harvard Educational Review,* 1947, *17,* 102–148.

Mowrer, O. H. *Learning theory and behavior.* New York: Wiley, 1960.

Murfin, F. L. *The relationship of fear to the CS-UCS interval in acquisition and the CS-duration in extinction.* Unpublished doctoral dissertation, University of Iowa, 1954.

Mylar, J. L., & Clement, P. W. Prediction and comparison of outcome in systematic desensitization and implosion. *Behaviour Research and Therapy,* 1972, *10,* 235–246.

Nathan, P. E., & Jackson, A. D. Behavior modification. In I. Winer (Ed.), *Clinical methods in psychology.* New York: Wiley Interscience, 1976.

Nau, S. D., Caputo, J. A., & Borkovec, T. D. The relationship between credibility of therapy rationale and the reduction of simulated anxiety, *Journal of Behavior Therapy and Experimental Psychiatry*, 1974, *5*, 129–133.

Naud, J., Boisvert, J., & Lamontagne, Y. Treatment of firearm phobia by flooding *in vivo* and motor activity: A case study. *Journal of Behavior Therapy and Experimental Psychiatry*, 1973, *4*, 407–409.

Nelson, F. Effects of two counter-conditioning procedures on the extinction of fear. *Journal of Comparative and Physiological Psychology*, 1966, *62*, 208–213.

Nelson, F. Effects of chlorpromazine on fear extinction. *Journal of Comparative and Physiological Psychology*, 1967, *64*, 469–498.

Nelson, F. Free versus forced exposure with two procedures for conditioning and measuring fear in the rat. *Journal of Comparative and Physiological Psychology*, 1969, *69*, 682–687.

Nesbitt, E. B. An escalator phobia overcome in one session of flooding *in vivo*. *Journal of Behavior Therapy and Experimental Psychiatry*, 1973, *4*, 405–406.

Newton, J. R., & Stein, L. I. Implosive therapy in alcoholism: Comparison with brief psychotherapy. *Quarterly Journal of Studies on Alcohol*, 1974, *35*, 1256–1265.

Nichols, M. P., & Zax, M. *Catharsis in psychotherapy*. New York: Gardner Press, 1977.

O'Donnell, J. M. Implosive therapy with hypnosis in the treatment of cancer phobia. *Psychotherapy: Theory, Research and Practice*, 1978, *10*, 47–48.

Ollendick, T. H., & Gruen, G. E. Treatment of a bodily injury phobia with implosive therapy. *Journal of Consulting and Clinical Psychology*, 1972, *38*, 389–393.

Olley, M., & McAllister, H. A comment on treatment analogues for phobic anxiety states. *Psychological Medicine*, 1974, *4*, 463–469.

Page, H. A. The facilitation of experimental extinction by response prevention as a function of the acquisition of a new response. *Journal of Comparative and Physiological Psychology*, 1955, *48*, 14–16.

Page, H. A., & Hall, J. F. Experimental extinction as a function of the prevention of a response. *Journal of Comparative and Physiological Psychology*, 1953, *46*, 33–34.

Parkinson, L., & Rachman, S. Are intrusive thoughts subject to habituation? *Behaviour Research and Therapy*, 1980, *18*, 409–418.

Pavlov, I. P. *Conditioned reflexes* [G. V. Anrep, Editor and translator] New York: Dover Publications, 1927. (Originally published, 1924.)

Pinto, R. A case of movement epilepsy with agoraphobia treated successfully by flooding. *British Journal of Psychiatry*, 1972, *121*, 287–288.

Polin, T. A. The effects of flooding and physical suppression of extinction technique on an anxiety-motivated avoidance locomotor response. *Journal of Psychology*, 1959, *47*, 235–245.

Prochaska, J. O. Symptom and dynamic cues in the implosive treatment of test anxiety. *Journal of Abonormal Psychology*, 1971, *77*, 133–142.

Rabavilas, A. D., & Boulougouris, J. C. Physiological accompaniment of ruminations, flooding and thought-stopping in obsessive patients. *Behaviour Research and Therapy*, 1974, *12*, 239–243.

Rabavilas, A. D., Boulougouris, J. C., & Stephanis, C. Duration of flooding sessions in the treatment of obsessive-compulsive patients. *Behaviour Research and Therapy*, 1976, *14*, 349–355

Rachman, S., Hodgson, R., & Marks, I. M. Treatment of chronic obsessive compulsive neurosis. *Behaviour Research and Therapy*, 1971, *9*, 237–247.

Rachman, S., Marks, I. M., & Hodgson, R. The treatment of obsessive-compulsive neurotics by modelling and flooding *in vivo*. *Behaviour Research and Therapy*, 1973, *11*, 463–471.

Rimm, D., & Bottrell, J. Four measures of visual imagination. *Behaviour Research and Therapy*, 1969, *7*, 63–69.

Rimm, D. C., & Masters, J. C. *Behavior therapy: Techniques and empirical findings.* New York: Academic Press, 1974.

Rosen, G. M. Is it really necessary to use mildly phobic analogue subjects? *Behavior Therapy*, 1975, *6*, 68–71.

Ross, S. M., & Proctor, S. Frequency and duration of hierarchy item exposure in a systematic desensitization analogue. *Behavior Research and Therapy*, 1973, *11*, 303–312.

Rubadeau, D. O., & Rubadeau, R. J. Treatment of a germ and crowd phobia by implosive therapy procedures *Canadian Journal of Behavioral Science*, 1972, 4, 249–252.

Sammah, M. Thought-stopping and flooding in a case of hallucinations, obsessions, and homicidal-suicidal behavior. *Journal of Behavior Therapy and Experimental Psychiatry*, 1975, *6*, 65–67.

Schiff, P., Smith, R. N., & Prochaska, J. Extinction of avoidance in rats as a function of duration and number of blocked trials. *Journal of Comparative and Physiological Psychology*, 1972, *81*, 356–359.

Shaw, P. A comparison of three behavior therapies in the treatment of social phobia. *British Journal of Psychiatry*, 1979, *134*, 620–623.

Shearman, R. W. Response-contingent CS termination in the extinction of avoidance learning. *Behaviour Research and Therapy*, 1970, *8*, 227–239.

Sheehan, P. W. A shortened form of Bett's questionnaire upon mental imagery. *Journal of Clinical Psychology*, 1967, *23*, 386–389.

Shepard, R. N. The mental image. *American Psychologist*, 1978, *33*, 125–137.

Sherrington, C. S. *The integrative action of the nervous system.* New Haven: Yale University Press, 1906.

Sherry, G. S., & Levine, B. A. An examination of procedural variables in flooding therapy. *Behavior Therapy*, 1980, *11*, 148–155.

Shipley, R. H. Extinction of conditioned fear in rats as a function of several parameters of CS exposure. *Journal of Comparative and Physiological Psychology*, 1974, *87*, 699–707.

Shipley, R. H. Implosive therapy: The technique. *Psychotherapy: Theory, Research and Practice*, 1979, *16*, 140–147.

Shipley, R. H. Behavioral management of acute anxiety and pain of stressful medical procedures. In P. A. Boudewyns & F. J. Keefe (Eds.), *Behavioral medicine in general medical practice.* New York: Addison-Wesley, 1982.

Shipley, R. H., & Boudewyns, P. A. How to overcome phobias: Self-control techniques. *Behavioral Medicine: Practical Information For Physicians.* 1979, *6*, 14–19.

Shipley, R. H., & Boudewyns, P. A. Flooding and implosive therapy: Are they harmful? *Behavior Therapy*, 1980, *11*, 503–508.

Shipley, R. H., Mock, L. A., & Levis, D. J. Effects of several response prevention procedures on activity, avoidance responding, and conditioned fear in rats. *Journal of Comparative and Physiological Psychology*, 1971, *77*, 256–270.

Shipley, R. H., Butt, J. H., Horwitz, B., & Farbry, J. Preparation for a stressful medical procedure: Effect of amount of stimulus preexposure and coping style. *Journal of Consulting and Clinical Psychology*, 1978, *46*, 499–507.

Shipley, R. H., Butt, J. H., & Horwitz, E. Preparations to re-experience a stressful medical examination: Effects of repetitious videotape exposure and coping style. *Journal of consulting and Clinical Psychology*, 1979, *47*, 485–492.

Silvestri, R. Implosive therapy treatment of emotionally disturbed retardates. *Journal of Consulting and Clinical Psychology*, 1977, *45*, 14–22.

Singer, J. L. *Imagery and daydream methods in psychotherapy and behavior modification.* New York: Academic Press, 1974.

Smith, R. E., & Sharpe, T. M. Treatment of school phobia with implosive therapy. *Journal of Consulting and Clinical Psychology*, 1970, *35*, 239-243.

Soloman, R. L. Punishment. *American Psychologist*, 1964, *19*, 237–253.

Solomon, R. L., & Wynne, L. C. Traumatic avoidance learning: The principles of anxiety conservation and partial irreversibility. *Psychological Review*, 1954, *61*, 353–385.

Solomon, R. L., Kamin, L. J., & Wynne, L. C. Traumatic avoidance learning: The outcomes of several extinction procedures with dogs. *Journal of Abnormal and Social Psychology*, 1953, *48*, 291–302.

Stambaugh, E. E. Audio-taped flooding in outpatient treatment of somatic complaints. *Journal of Behavior Therapy and Experimental Psychiatry*, 1977, *8*, 173–176.

Stampfl, T. G. *Implosive therapy: A learning theory derived psychodynamic therapeutic technique.* Paper presented at Colloquium of the University of Illinois, 1961.

Stampfl, T. G. Implosive therapy: An emphasis on covert stimulation. In D. J. Levis (Ed.), *Learning approaches to therapeutic behavior change.* Chicago: Aldine, 1970.

Stampfl, T. G., & Levis, D. J. Implosive therapy. In R. M. Jurjevich (Ed.), *Handbook of direct and behavior psychotherapies.* Englewood Cliffs, N.J.: Prentice-Hall, 1966.

Stampfl, T. G., & Levis, D. J. Essentials of implosive therapy: A learning-theory-based psychodynamic behavioral therapy. *Journal of Abnormal Psychology*, 1967, *72*, 496–503.

Stampfl, T. G., & Levis, D. J. Learning Theory: An aid to dynamic therapeutic practice. In L. D. Eron & R. Callahan (Eds.), *The relation of theory to practice in psychotherapy.* Chicago: Aldine, 1969.

Stern, R. S. Obsessive thoughts: The problem of therapy. *British Journal of Psychiatry*, 1978, *133*, 200–205.

Stern, R. S., & Marks, I. M. Brief and prolonged flooding: A comparison in agoraphobic patients. *Archives of General Psychiatry*, 1973, *28*, 270–276.

Stone, N. M., & Borkovec, T. D. The paradoxical effect of brief CS exposure on analogue phobic subjects. *Behaviour Research and Therapy*, 1975, *13*, 51–54.

Strosahl, K. D., & Ascough, J. C. Clinical uses of mental imagery: Experimental foundations, theoretical misconceptions, and research issues. *Psychological Bulletin*, 1981, *89*, 422–438.

Switras, J. E. An alternate-form instrument to assess vividness and controllability of mental imagery in seven modalities. *Perceptual and Motor Skills*, 1978, *46*, 379–384.

Taub, J., Taylor, P., Smith, M., Kelley, K., Becker, B., & Reid, L. Methods of deconditioning persisting avoidance: Drugs as adjuncts to response prevention. *Physiological Psychology*, 1977, *5*, 67–72.

Teasdale, J. D., Walsh, P. A., Lancashire, M., & Mathews, A. M. Group exposure for agoraphobics: A replication study. *British Journal of Psychiatry*, 1977, *30*, 186–193.

Testa, T. J. Comments on: Residual fear of the conditioned stimulus as a function of response prevention after avoidance or classical defensive conditioning in the rat. *Journal of Experimental Psychology*, 1976, *2*, 163–168.

Thomas, M., & Rapp, M. Physiological, behavioral and cognitive changes resulting from flooding in a monosymptomatic phobic. *Behaviour Research and Therapy*, 1977, *15*, 304–306.

Trudel, G. The effects of instruction and level of fear. *Behaviour Research and Therapy*, 1979, *17*, 113–118.

Turner, S. M., Hersen, M., Bellack, A. S. & Wells, K. C. Behavioral treatment of obsessive-compulsive neurosis. *Behaviour Research and Therapy*, 1978, *17*, 95–106.

Van Egeren, L. F., Feather, B. W., & Hein, P. L. Desensitization of phobics: Some psychophysiological propositions. *Psychophysiology*, 1971, *8*, 213–228.

Wallace, J., & Scobie, S. Avoidance extinction in goldfish. *Learning and Motivation*, 1977, *8*, 18–38.

Waters, W., & McDonald, D. Autonomic response to auditory, visual, and imagined stimuli in a systematic desensitization context. *Behaviour Research and Therapy*, 1973, *11*, 577–585.

Watson, J. P., Gaind, R., & Marks, I. M. Prolonged exposure: A rapid treatment for phobias. *British Medical Journal*, 1971, *1*, 13–15.

Watson, J. P., & Marks, I. M. Relevant and irrelevant fear in flooding—A cross-over study of phobic patients. *Behavior Therapy*, 1971, *2*, 275–293.

Watson, J. P., Mullett, G. E., & Pillay, H. The effects of prolonged exposure to phobic situations upon agoraphobic patients treated in groups. *Behaviour Research and Therapy*, 1973, *11*, 531.

Weeks, C. *Simple, effective treatment of agoraphobia.* New York: Hawthorn Books, 1970.

Whitehead, W. E., Blackwell, B., & Robinson, A. Effects of diazepam on phobic avoidance behavior and phobic anxiety. *Biological Psychiatry*, 1978, *13*, 59–64.

Whitehead, W. E., Robinson, A., Blackwell, B., & Stutz, R. M. Flooding treatment of phobias: Does chronic diazepam increase effectiveness? *Journal of Behavior Therapy and Experimental Psychiatry*, 1978, *9*, 219–225.

Wijesinghe, B. A vomiting phobia overcome by one session of flooding with hypnosis. *Journal of Behavior Therapy and Experimental Psychiatry*, 1974, *5*, 169–170.

Wilson, A. E., Smith, F. J. Counterconditioning therapy using free association: A pilot study. *Journal of Abnormal Psychology*, 1968, *73*, 474–478.

Wilson, G. T. Counterconditioning versus forced exposure in extinction of avoidance responding and conditioned fear in rats. *Journal of Comparative and Physiological Psychology*, 1973, *83*, 105–114.

Wilson, G. T., & Davison, G. C. Processes of fear reduction in systematic desensitization: Animal studies. *Psychological Bulletin*, 1971, *76*, 1–14.

Wolpe, J. *Psychotherapy by reciprocal inhibition.* Stanford: Stanford University Press, 1958.

Wolpe, J. *The practice of behavior therapy.* New York: Pergamon Press, 1969.

Yule, W., Sacks, B., & Hersov, L. Successful flooding treatment of a noise phobia in an eleven-year-old. *Journal of Behavior Therapy and Experimental Psychiatry*, 1974, *5*, 209–211.

Zimmerman, J. If it's what's inside that counts, why not count it? Self-recording of feelings and treatment by "self-implosition". *Psychological Record*, 1975, *25*, 3–16.

Zitrin, C. M., Klein, D. F., & Woerner, M. G. Treatment of agoraphobia with group exposure *in vivo* and imipramine. *Archives of General Psychiatry*, 1980, *37*, 63–72.

Zitrin, C. M., Klein, D. F., Lindeman, C., Tobak, P., Rock, M., Koplan, J., & Ganz, V. H. Comparison of short-term treatment regimens in phobic patients: A preliminary report. In R. L. Spitzer & D. F. Klein (Eds.), *Evaluation of psychological therapies.* Baltimore: Johns Hopkins University Press, 1976.

Zitrin, C. M. Combined pharmacological and psychological treatment for phobias. In M. Mavissakalian, & D. H. Barlow (Eds.), *Phobia.* New York: Guilford Press, 1981.

AUTHOR INDEX

SUBJECT INDEX